GOD'S Rx

for INNER HEALING

JAMES P. GILLS, MD

SILOAM

Most Charisma House Book Group products are available at special quantity discounts for bulk purchase for sales promotions, premiums, fund-raising, and educational needs. For details, call us at (407) 333-0600 or visit our website at www.charismahouse.com.

God's Rx for Inner Healing by James P. Gills, MD
Published by Siloam
Charisma Media/Charisma House Book Group
600 Rinehart Road, Lake Mary, Florida 32746

Visit the author's website at www.stlukeseye.com.

Library of Congress Cataloging-in-Publication Data

Names: Gills, James P., 1934- author.
Title: God's Rx for inner healing / by James P. Gills.
Description: Lake Mary, Florida : Siloam, [2019] | Includes bibliographical
    references.
Identifiers: LCCN 2019007366 (print) | LCCN 2019010313 (ebook) | ISBN
    9781629996424 (e-book) | ISBN 9781629996417 (trade paper) | ISBN
    9781629996424 (ebk.)
Subjects: LCSH: Spiritual healing--Christianity.
Classification: LCC BT732.5 (ebook) | LCC BT732.5 .G55 2019 (print) |
DDC
    248.8/6--dc23
LC record available at https://lccn.loc.gov/2019007366

ISBN: 978-1-62999-641-7
E-book ISBN: 978-1-62999-642-4

Portions of this book were previously published by Siloam as *God's
Prescription for Healing*, ISBN 0-88419-947-9, copyright © 2004 and by
Charisma House as *Resting in His Redemption*, ISBN 978-1-61638-349-7,
copyright © 2011.

This publication is translated in Spanish under the title *La prescripción
de Dios para la salud interna*, copyright © 2019 by James P. Gills, MD,
published by Casa Creación, a Charisma Media company. All rights
reserved.

19 20 21 22 23 — 987654321
Printed in the United States of America

CONTENTS

INTRODUCTION

ONCE KNEW A wonderful gentleman who lived a long, peaceful life so filled with joy that all who knew him loved him. They sometimes expressed their wonder at the glow of peace and joy that radiated from him and the gorgeous smile that lit up his face when he greeted them. He had a way of making each person he saw feel special. Even in times of crisis he reflected the peace of God in his demeanor and was obviously full of joy.

My friend was often asked why he seemed so happy. He would smile broadly and say that his communion with God was his source of happiness. When pressed to explain, he shared that throughout his life he made a practice of reading the Scriptures several hours a day and praying diligently in pursuit of an intimate relationship with His lovely Lord. He had learned that getting to know God was much sweeter than anything this natural life had to offer. And in turn his communion with God made his life much sweeter.

He added that his continual fellowship with the Lord gave him a profound sense of belonging to God and of being deeply loved by Him. That divine love filled his heart with peace and joy. As a result he lived his life sharing the love of God with others. He had learned to appreciate and value each person the way God does. And in seeking God's heart, he escaped the temptations of fear, anxiety, anger, and other negative emotional responses to the harmful experiences of our troubled world.

In stark contrast to my friend's exuberant joy, the wife of this godly man was constantly atwitter, worried about this, concerned about that. Her countenance did not reflect peace but anxiety and unrest. She was known to be critical of others, even fellow believers in Christ.

This unhappy woman did not understand what scientific studies show: in many people these negative attitudes are some of the telltale signs of harmful past experiences, which have left unresolved and unhealed inner wounds. Often without realizing it, people can carry these inner wounds throughout their lives, never finding freedom from the harmful emotional aftermath of their painful past.

Though she said she was a Christian, my friend's wife lived as if she were solely responsible for life's every moment. She did not take time to pursue God as her husband did. She did not seek God's rest and joy for herself, though she was a constant witness to the fruit of that divine relationship in the demeanor of her husband. At the time of his death, they had been married sixty years. Yet his wife had never received the comfort her husband offered her or the love he wanted to share with her.

For her, being a Christian was more of an outward appearance. It was based on religious actions that belied her inner anxiety as she attempted to control every aspect of her life. In her constant state of unrest she never truly experienced the intimate love relationship with God her husband enjoyed. As a result she forfeited the comfort of intimate communion with her husband as well as with her God.

Unfortunately this negative, anxious behavior of my friend's wife seems common in many people, even professing Christians. They do not reflect the radiant peace, joy, and loving character displayed by my friend. In his constant pursuit of God, my friend discovered the purpose for living: to totally abandon ourselves to Christ, yielding to His loving control, so that we become filled with His love and reflect His character of love, joy, and peace.

Throughout his life my friend gave of himself to others—and not just his money but the compassion and love of Christ. He blessed many people with the peace and joy he received from his Lord by resting in His redemption.

I wrote an entire book about resting in God's redemption, and some of the content I have provided in this book was originally published in that book. For the purpose of this book we will focus on an understanding of rest, faith, and forgiveness, all of which are essential to inner healing of deep wounds and negative attitudes. I encourage you to pick up a copy of *Resting in His Redemption* if you would like to go further in your study of this concept.

There are countless ways we may be ill, out of balance, and suffering. Likewise, then, there are numberless ways we may be healed through God's wonderful "prescription" for our healing. God's wisdom and mercy are unfathomable. He desires to restore balance and harmony within our entire being, including our inner selves. In this book we will examine some key causes of our distress of mind and emotions and consider God's wonderful provision for our inner healing.

Meant to help us peer more deeply at the heart of God and His care of us, this book can reinforce faith for those who believe in Christ as their loving Savior. It can be a source of support for those who are suffering and need healing in their own lives or want to see healing in the lives of loved ones. In some cases of deep emotional wounds or severe past trauma, it may be necessary to seek professional help, such as a Christian counselor. As you read, ask God for the wisdom to know the best course of action you should take on your journey to inner healing and complete wholeness of body, mind, and spirit.

CHAPTER 1

DESIGNED FOR
COMMUNION WITH GOD

B ECAUSE WE ARE designed by our Creator to live in sweet communion with God, it follows that we are designed to enjoy inner health and wholeness, mentally and emotionally. We are meant to live a life of peace and satisfaction as we pursue the purpose for which we were born. We are not intended to suffer the pain of depression, anxiety, fear, hopelessness, and other negative mindsets and emotions that plagues so many people, even Christians.

Perhaps you or someone you love is living in the misery described here and in spite of sincere pursuits—medical or otherwise—has not been able to find peace and freedom of heart and mind. In the pages of this small book you will learn many practical ways people have found hope, peace, and healing from deep wounds, restoring their lives to the fulfillment and satisfaction for which they were born. Their stories and the evidence of those principles and practices that bring inner healing to wounded hearts will help you to evaluate your life situation and to find relief from your pain as well.

In this chapter we will define some terms and establish God's loving desire and wonderful plan for your inner health. It is important to know His "story" and love for mankind and how He wants it to become your "story." Simply stated, to receive inner healing that results in an inward state of joy and peace and hope for the future is to receive the love of God personally, to be restored to right relationship with Him. Yet there are practical ways to learn how you can make God's desire for your inner wholeness become a reality in your life. Then you will be able to make decisions, as others have, to be a joyful participant in God's story.

When you enter into a personal relationship with God, it is the desire of God's heart that you be filled with delight and enjoyment and enter into the *mystery* of a divine romance with Him. Enjoying God means living our lives filled with His divine love and free from fear, doubt, worry, anger, and other negative mindsets. In short, it means *resting in Him*. This intimate relationship with God is not found in simply assenting to religious creeds and following religious traditions. The Scriptures teach that when we learn to place our faith in Christ, we can enter His divine rest: "For we who have believed do enter that rest" (Heb. 4:3).

In contrast, man-centered religion demands self-effort that "rests" in its own self-righteous works. Trying to do good things and follow religious traditions is not the same as entering into intimate relationship with God through faith in Him. Even good things such as giving and prayer are reduced to religious self-effort if we do not learn to enter into the spiritual rest Christ's redemption promises to us. Emotional and mental turmoil are not eased or conquered through religious practices and traditions. Only as you apply the spiritual principles and other practical applications of the truth we will discuss here can you make God's love story yours.

Many Christians have not fully understood that redemption through faith in Christ offers them the enjoyment of His indescribable peace, joy, and divine rest—the mystery of divine romance with God. We all get a measure of this at conversion, but too often we lose sight it. We must return to our first love. This kind of communion with God is possible as we learn to yield to the Holy Spirit and seek Him to guide us into all truth (John 16:13). He will show us "the path of life" (Ps. 16:11) and lead us into the restful peace and joy Christ offers to those who choose to abide in Him. More than just physical rest, the heart of every person yearns for this intimate spiritual communion with God.

Are you living a life of delightful, intimate relationship with your Lord, basking in the pool of His grace as displayed in the life of the friend I mentioned in the introduction? Are you abandoned to resting in the river of His love that fills you with peace even in the face of difficult circumstances? Is the Holy Spirit filling you with God's divine love for others?

Or do you find yourself easily triggered to overreact emotionally? Do you hold grudges and constantly justify yourself in your mind with the wrongs that have been done to you? Do you see bad patterns in your life that tend to repeat themselves, such as continuously burning bridges with employers or struggling to establish healthy relationships with family and friends? These are signs of unresolved inner wounds that disturb your inner peace and lead to weariness, unhappiness, insecurity, and depression.

If left unresolved, these wounds from your past will rob you of the enjoyment of communion with God that He intended. They will prevent you from sharing the genuine love you were meant to give and receive in your relationships with other people. The fact is, it is possible to think you are living the Christian life as it was intended and never truly experience the joy, peace, and inner healing found only in learning to rest in His loving redemption.

UNDERSTANDING REST

As a few more terms are defined, you will be able to identify what your mindset is concerning life as God intended you to enjoy it in a state of inner wholeness. An example is *rest*. Just seeing the word itself may help you locate the life struggles that rob you of that desirable peace and tranquility of spirit, mind, and body. Thinking of rest may bring to mind your favorite way to relax, kick back, and recreate. Hopefully, contemplating the wonderful reality of rest stirs a longing in your heart to experience the inner peace, serenity, and sense of well-being that only God's divine rest offers you.

Usually when we speak of rest, we are referring to resting our bodies and our minds from the rigors of everyday living, working, and other responsibilities. That is actually the primary meaning of the word *rest*. However, while physical rest is vital to our well-being, it is not the profound essence of rest we crave most as human beings. Physical cessation from activity alone will not bring the rest to our hearts and minds that we were created to enjoy.

A more profound definition of *rest* is inner "peace of mind or spirit."[1] It is this sublime spiritual rest that we yearn for most. Without experiencing true spiritual rest, we cannot receive healing from deep wounds and disappointments of our past; without spiritual rest we cannot find true happiness or fulfillment in life, no matter how hard or where we search for it. Even our physical rest is compromised without our discovering the source of true spiritual rest.

THE "DOOR" TO SPIRITUAL REST

This divine spiritual rest we crave is a result of first coming to Christ and accepting His redemption by placing our faith in Him. That is only the first step into our relationship with Him. Many Christians fail to live in all that Christ's redemption promises them because they do not seek Him as a result of a deep spiritual conviction that leads them to cultivate a profound personal relationship with Him. Receiving Christ's forgiveness for our sin restores us to relationship to God, which Adam and Eve lost through their disobedience. Jesus taught that we "must be born again" (John 3:7) to receive His gift of eternal life, which He purchased for our redemption through His death on the cross. Confessing our sinful state and asking for cleansing through His precious blood grants us entrance into personal peace with God: "Therefore being justified by faith, we have peace with God through our Lord Jesus Christ" (Rom. 5:1, KJV).

Yet that is just the beginning of our restoration to profound spiritual rest of body, mind, and spirit. As in any human friendship, it is as we spend time with each other, share hearts, and build trust that we forge a profound heart relationship with Christ. As we continually seek the Holy Spirit to reveal His love, His will, and His purpose to us, we receive Christ's divine healing for our wounded hearts. Spending time with Him by reading His Word, praying, and waiting on Him forges the strength and depth of relationship with the power to ultimately restore us to divine rest in every area of our lives. As we cultivate that intimate relationship with Christ, we learn to enjoy God and glorify Him in all we do.

UNDERSTANDING MANKIND'S CHIEF END

Saint Augustine, the renowned early church father, opened his famous theological treatise *Confessions* by describing the chief end of mankind, the ultimate purpose for creation:

> Thou has formed us for Thyself, and our hearts are restless till they find rest in Thee....Oh! how shall I find rest in Thee? Who will send Thee into my heart to inebriate it, that I may forget my woes, and embrace Thee, my only good?...Alas! alas! Tell me of Thy compassion, O Lord my God, what Thou art to me. "Say unto my soul, I am thy salvation." So speak that I may hear. Behold, Lord, the ears of my heart are before Thee; open Thou them, and "say unto my soul, I am thy salvation." When I hear, may I run and

lay hold on Thee. Hide not Thy face from me. Let me die, lest I die, if only I may see Thy face.[2]

Our Creator-Redeemer formed us to experience the bliss of His love by living in perpetual communion with Him. Have you considered this most profound aspect of your need for true spiritual rest? For peace of mind? For the divine communion with God that Saint Augustine cried out for? Have you considered that God alone is your source for ultimate healing from your painful past and for your enjoyment, your contentment, and the fulfillment of your destiny in life?

Or are you one of many who are busy just trying to find a way to enjoy a little physical rest and recreation? A little psychological relief in your favorite escape? Just plodding through each day, trying to be in control of your life, hoping for a little less grief tomorrow? Relief is ill hoped for unless you pursue the purpose for which you were created: "to glorify God, and to enjoy him for ever."[3]

I believe it is the longing for this true spiritual rest, so desperately needed and so little understood, that drives millions of people to the pharmacy in search of medications they hope will artificially induce the relief they seek. Others may try to escape their painful past and lack of peace through the use of illicit drugs, alcohol, or other equally harmful and inadequate means.

GOD'S HEART FOR MANKIND

According to the Scriptures, God created mankind on the sixth day of His creative work, during which He called into being the universe and all of creation as we know it. The sixth day was the last day of God's work of creation. What we learn next from the Scriptures may seem a little strange to us: after six days of creative work God *rested* (Gen. 2:2).

One can hardly deduce from those words God was tired after His work of creation. An omnipotent God would certainly not have needed to "recuperate" from His magnificent work of creation, would He? Yet God reserved a day of rest, a time for ceasing from all activity, to celebrate the work He had done. He blessed the seventh day because He rested from all His work (v. 3).

Later God called that day of rest the Sabbath (Hebrew, *shabbath*), which is from a word that means "to repose…desist from exertion…celebrate."[4] Have you considered what significance there might be in the fact that mankind's first full day of life was the day of God's *shabbath*? Rest. Celebration. What a lovely way for mankind, God's jewel of creation, to begin life in the presence of the Creator!

It is as we are restored to relationship with God through Christ's redemption that the purity of that original spiritual environment of rest will allow us to fulfill the true works for which He created us. Rather than our self-righteous efforts that are sometimes motivated by a desire to make a name for ourselves, our restoration to God will allow us to discover the true meaning of life as He intended. The New Testament confirms: "For we are his workmanship, created in Christ Jesus unto good works, which God hath before ordained that we should walk in them" (Eph. 2:10, KJV). Unless we fully yield our lives to Christ, we can never know the good works God has ordained us to accomplish. And all our religious effort will result only in a sense of pride for what we did or in weariness in our spent energies; it will not fill us with the peace and joy that come from fulfilling God's will for our lives.

The Book of Genesis tells us that God created mankind in His image (Gen. 1:27). And the Scriptures teach us that "God is Spirit" (John 4:24). That spiritual image of God within us continually desires to experience *shabbath*: the rest of God. When God made a requirement for mankind to keep a *shabbath* as a day of rest from all labor (Exod. 20:10–11), it was to give us a temporal, physical rest during which we can be refreshed in His spiritual rest.

It is that spiritual rest of living in continual harmony with our Creator and Savior for which our souls yearn most deeply. We were created for intimate relationship with God. Without experiencing His continual presence in our lives, we are doomed to unrest and unhappiness. God is not only a Spirit; "God is love" (1 John 4:8). The entire message of the Bible reveals that the purpose of God in creating mankind was to have a family—sons and daughters—with whom He could have fellowship and share His heart of love.

The great, loving heart of God designed mankind to know happiness and fulfillment only through an intimate relationship with Him. And in our restoration to Him through our salvation through Christ, He wants us to celebrate all of life with Him as He ordained it to be. According to God's original plan, the divine mystery and romance of His love were to be consummated in each human heart as they lived life in the presence of God. In that sacred relationship mankind would rest in absolute safety and bliss with their Creator. They would be continually receiving the love of God and accepting all of His gifts with joy—that was the infinite, loving heart of God for mankind, the jewel of His creation. In that relationship they would experience wholeness in their inner being and enjoy the fulfillment of love, joy, and peace our hearts crave today. And in their continual communion with God, mankind would learn to walk in the divinely ordained works God had prepared for them.

GOD'S PLAN FOR REDEMPTION

Unfortunately that first couple failed to follow God's glorious plan for mankind to enjoy communion with God. And they contaminated the entire human race when they decided to live independently from God and to be in charge of their own lives. God turned man over to the consequences of his sin of disobedience to God's commands. Physical death entered the scene; spiritual death, i.e., separation from God, became an eternal reality; and there was no hope of redemption to be found in man's own efforts.

Yet even in that tragic scene God pursued Adam and Eve and initiated the promise of His plan of redemption for mankind. He spoke to the serpent, identified as the devil, who had deceived the couple into disobeying God, and promised, "I will put enmity between you and the woman, and between your seed and her Seed; He shall bruise your head, and you shall bruise His heel" (Gen. 3:15). Theologians call this verse the protevangelium, meaning the first mention of God's promise to redeem mankind back to Himself through the Seed of the woman, referring to Christ's redemption at Calvary. For thousands of years God pursued mankind, making covenants with His chosen instruments who had a part in fulfilling His redemptive promise.

God calls mankind to live in His love and to seek relationship with Him. That is the true nature of satisfying love—a relationship based on fulfilled desire, not on keeping rules. The mystery of love involves a reciprocation of two hearts that cherish each other and want to live in harmony together. Out of that love they are willing to accept any conditions placed on the relationship to avoid disrupting the harmony they enjoy. We long to please Him and fulfill our purpose for life by walking in the works He ordained for us.

When Adam and Eve chose to disobey God, they disrupted the harmony of that divine romance. As a result they lost the source of the divine rest they craved, which was to be found only in a satisfying fellowship with their Creator. When that happened, God began the long, arduous task of redeeming mankind, calling us back to the blissful rest for which we were created. Down through the centuries of mankind's existence God continually reached down to us, working His plan of redemption.

REDEMPTION DEFINED

Before we can truly experience the inner healing that comes from resting in His redemption, we need to understand the significance of the word. *Redemption* means "the act of delivering from sin or saving from evil." It also signifies "the act of purchasing back something previously sold."[5] When Adam and Eve "sold out" to the devil's lie that by disobeying God, they would become as gods, it became necessary for God to purchase back lost mankind from the clutches of evil. He had to redeem mankind through the death of His Son, Jesus Christ so we could once again become sons and daughters of God who would walk in sweet fellowship with Him.

In the scope of this small book we cannot trace the loving heart of the Father as He pursued mankind through the centuries. However, we must understand that He culminated His plan of redemption when He sent His Son, Jesus, to save us from our sins. The initial act of receiving Christ's sacrifice for our sin is the only way we can be restored to God's original purpose for mankind. It is our only hope of experiencing His wholeness—His righteousness, peace, and joy for our lives—as we cultivate the intimate relationship with Him that He originally intended. As we look briefly at God's pursuit of mankind, I believe it will help you appreciate at a new depth the great love of God for each of us.

DIVINE REST IN THE OLD TESTAMENT

The essence of the entire message of the over thirty thousand verses in the Bible is this reality of enjoying an intimate relationship with God. It is this central truth of the Scriptures that leads our sin-sick souls back to the profound spiritual rest in which we were created to live. That was God's desire even for Old Testament saints who lived before the victory of Calvary yet walked in God's revealed precepts.

The fall of mankind into sin through Adam and Eve's disobedience did not catch God by surprise. God planned the redemption of mankind before the creation of the world. The Scriptures refer to Christ as "the Lamb slain from the foundation of the world" (Rev. 13:8). The essence of the Old Testament is the story of God enacting this divine plan of redemption through His prophets, priests, and kings who helped guide His people back to His rest.

For example, when God called Israel to be a nation, He redeemed them through the hand of Moses from their cruel bondage to Pharaoh. You remember the provision He made to spare the firstborn of Israel by having the people place the blood of a lamb on the doorposts of their homes. As they did so in obedience to His word, they were saying, in effect, "We rest in God's redemption." They trusted in His word to them that He would protect them from the scourge of death that was coming to judge the Egyptians.

And He did pass over those homes where the blood of the lamb was applied. God instituted the feast of Passover for Israel to celebrate that deliverance from destruction. As they celebrated this Passover feast, they were acknowledging God's power to bring them to the doorway of faith as a nation.

When God gave Moses detailed instructions in the wilderness to build a tabernacle, He was once again seeking a way to dwell with His people, to be near them, protect them, and give them His rest. God longed to commune with them, so He told Moses to make a mercy seat, a golden lid over the ark of the covenant, where the blood of the atonement would be sprinkled. And God said He would meet with His high priest there. It would be the dwelling place of God's glory where He would speak to mankind. There He would show them mercy and let them experience relationship with Him. He would speak to them there, guiding and directing them and giving them power over their enemies.

After the tabernacle was built, the Israelites marched toward Canaan, the Promised Land, where God said they would live in rest, peace, and abundance. He promised to be with them to conquer the enemies that dwelled in the land. However, when they arrived, they realized there were giants in the land.

They also found that the cities there had high, thick walls, so the people were afraid they could not conquer them.

Joshua and Caleb reminded the people that God was with them and would help them conquer the land He had promised to give to them. But the people refused to trust God's word. Because they did not believe the word of God to them, they were forced to wander in the wilderness for the rest of their lives. Everyone of that generation who gave in to fear instead of grabbing the promise in faith died wandering in that wilderness. Only then did the second generation get to march into the Promised Land.

The only exceptions to this sad fate were Joshua and Caleb, men from the first generation who believed the Lord's promise and declared it to the people. Joshua led Israel into the Promised Land. He prepared them for battle, and they began to conquer the enemies in the land. Caleb asked for a mountain in the Promised Land and was granted the strength to conquer it. Joshua and Caleb were victorious because they chose to trust in the promises of God and to rest in His provision.

Though the Israelites had come out of Egypt, their miraculous redemption from that four hundred years of captivity did not automatically lead them into an understanding of resting in God's love, power, and redemption. Because they refused to trust God to give them all He had promised, He would not let them enter the Promised Land of His rest. The New Testament teaches that their unbelief, their lack of faith, kept them from receiving the rest He had promised to them.

THE CALL TO SPIRITUAL REST

God repeatedly called men and women in the Old Testament to enter into His rest. He wanted them to experience the intimate relationship with Him as their Creator-Redeemer that He had ordained from the beginning. King David, also known as "the sweet psalmist of Israel" (2 Sam. 23:1), understood that God's redemptive rest was a reality for those who would seek Him through prayer and meditation on His Word. (See Psalm 37:5, 7.)

The Book of Psalms declares, "For the LORD hath chosen Zion; he hath desired it for his habitation. This is my rest for ever: here will I dwell; for I have desired it" (Ps. 132:13–14, KJV). God revealed His choice to dwell with mankind and let them enjoy the spiritual rest of His presence.

God delights to be our God, our heavenly Father. And He longs to dwell among us and give us His rest. If God is content to dwell with us and let us hear His voice, then it is foolish for us not to be content to rest in His love through learning to commune with Him in personal prayer and worship.

When Jesus came to the earth to become our Redeemer, He confirmed the Father's desire for intimate fellowship with us: "If a man love me, he will keep my words: and my Father will love him, and *we will come unto him, and make our abode with him*" (John 14:23, KJV, emphasis added).

As we discussed, since the moment sin entered the world through Adam and Eve's disobedience, God has been working His plan to redeem, to buy back, all that He lost in not having sons and daughters. He is determined to buy back as well our rest, peace, and joy in experiencing the mystery of the divine romance for which He created mankind originally. He has made it possible through Christ's sacrifice for our sins not only for us to experience total well-being in our lives on earth but also to live with Him eternally in absolute bliss.

The saints in the Old Testament had trials in their lives that sometimes distracted them and kept them from entering the rest of God. The psalmist knew that there was only one thing to do when that happened: "Return to your rest, O my soul, for the LORD has dealt bountifully with you" (Ps. 116:7). Likewise, when we get distracted from focusing on living in God's presence, we need to recognize why we say "I am uneasy," "I am restless," "I am trusting in my own efforts," or "I am worrying and full of fear." And we need to say to ourselves, as the psalmist did, "I must go back to the wonderful place of rest I have found in God's love through Christ's redemption. There my heart will be at peace and God's Spirit will comfort me and strengthen me and give me all I need to confront life's situations, whether past or present."

Many years after the kingdom of Israel became a divided kingdom, God was still reaching out to His wayward people. Through prophets such as Isaiah and Jeremiah, God called His people back to His rest. Their constant refusal to return to God's rest did not deter His loving heart from pursuing them. The entire Old Testament is filled with God's voice summoning His people to respond to His call of love, to return to His paths where they would find His rest. Many times they refused to hear the heart of God. Yet He continued to reveal His desire to redeem them, to reinstate His love relationship with them.

Through the centuries, God continued to reveal His love to mankind through the prophets. He gave them hope and prepared His people to receive His Son, Jesus Christ, who would offer the ultimate atonement for the sin of the whole world. Christ would personally atone for every person's sin against God. He would redeem us back to our rightful place of resting in His redemption. It is up to each one of us to receive the wonderful redemption love that God offers to us. As we do, we begin our journey into His rest, which will result in our inner healing and wholeness.

DISCUSSION ❦ QUESTIONS

Is prayer essential to our communion with God? Explain.

....

....

....

....

As a Christian, can you experience divine peace and a sense of well-being without resting in His redemption? Explain.

....

....

....

According to Saint Augustine, our hearts are restless until they find their rest in God. Do you agree? Why or why not?

....

....

....

....

CHAPTER 2

WHAT IS
INNER HEALING?

HAT WAS THE pattern for mankind's inner healing and wholeness that God intended when He created mankind? How do we know what is "normal" for us to feel and think as human beings created in God's image? How does our redemption through Christ affect our mindsets and negative emotions?

Humans are so much more than clumps of tissue and the results of their labor. We are not simply physical entities as codfish and fir trees are. We are physical, mental, emotional, and spiritual beings. All aspects of our exceptionally designed bodies are integrated into a unified whole, which is greater than the sum of its parts. The amazing completeness of the entire person mirrors this life-giving principle. And yet for many people, painful experiences from the past keep them trapped in a prison of negative emotions, such as anxiety, fear, anger, worry, depression, and more. Healing these emotional wounds is vital if you want to experience wholeness and the fullness of everything God has purposed for your life. So how does healing register in your inner experience?

Wholeness for a person means balance and communication between body, mind, emotions, and spirit. Wholeness and balance at the mental and spiritual levels are proven to affect the capacity of your body to heal physically. Additionally, as a thinking, feeling creation of the Creator, you also have need of mental and spiritual healing when balance has been overturned in those areas as well. What is required for this healing of mind and spirit? What is God's prescription for your inner healing then?

God's Word tells us that we need to be transformed in our thinking (Rom. 12:2) and aligned to the mind of Christ (Phil. 2:5) in order to be the recipient of all the health and wholeness He offers those who yield their lives to Him. It takes full surrender to Christ to engage in this integration of body, soul, and spirit that results in wholeness. For example, we need to yield our will to God, as Christ did in Gethsemane: "Not My will, but Yours, be done" (Luke 22:42).

This denial of self with its selfish desires and goals presents you to God as a holy, pleasing, and available recipient of all He is. It is the key to receiving His life of continual healing—health and wholeness—spiritually as well as physically. He made us to live in harmony with Him in order for our entire being to run smoothly. His main purpose for such costly redemption was to draw us into the intimate fellowship with Him for which we were designed.

When we speak of physical health and healing, we are referring to maintaining or reacquiring balance within the body by adhering to required guidelines that the body's design dictates. You align yourself with God's purpose for your physical health by accepting the stewardship of your temple, in which He dwells. When we speak of balance in hearts and minds, you may think of it as realignment with the spiritual principles and precepts of thinking and feeling for which you were created. Having "the mind of Christ" (1 Cor. 2:16) and yielding your heart to receive His divine love is the pathway to inner healing. When you are firmly established on that pathway, filling your mind and heart with His Word and cultivating intimate relationship with Him, you are on a journey to fulfill God's design and plan for your inner healing and wholeness.

The Word clearly teaches that mentally you must seek to have the mind of Christ (Phil. 2:5). That involves yielding to the Holy Spirit for His help to keep you thinking positive thoughts, having a hopeful perspective, and rejoicing with great feelings of thankfulness. Spiritually you must have God's Holy Spirit reigning in every part of your being. And by focusing on eternal life rather than on your temporal circumstances, you are aligning yourself with God and His purposes for your life, i.e. inner wholeness (2 Cor. 4:16–18). Inner healing is the healing of mind and spirit. This inner healing will also strengthen the health of your body. Our capacity to receive inner healing is determined by our divine design in creation.

MIND AND BODY—BODY AND MIND

Intuitively, you are aware that you are not comprised of "divided" portions of body, mind, and spirit. Each of these areas of your life is profoundly connected, each a part of a singularity, and therefore each deeply influences the others. Those influences are more profound than you may know, however. Science is just now teasing out the details of the depth of the relationships between body, mind, and spirit. For example, recent research indicates that emotional pain excites the same parts of the brain as strongly as physical pain.[1]

Some illnesses heal under the energies of the body's natural systems. Some require medical intervention, while the healing of others can be accomplished through diet, exercise, and lifestyle changes. And yet other illness can be attributed to one's mental and spiritual state. Errant emotions, fears, and anxieties can kill. The realignment of your inner self can assist in restoring your overall well-being.

Numerous studies have now pointed out the weighty influence of the mind-body connection. We are being increasingly informed about the role of depression, loneliness, unhappiness, fear, and anger in the development and prolongation of diseases such as cancer, heart disease, diabetes, and asthma.[2] The mind refers to the complete array of mental functions "related to thinking, mood, and purposive behavior. The mind is generally seen as deriving from activities in the brain but displaying emergent properties, such as consciousness."[3]

Typically, we think of the mind as centered in the brain. Scientific research indicates that our thoughts and feelings influence the body through two primary channels, the nervous system and the circulatory system.[4] The brain, as the center of the nervous system, sends and receives electrical impulses from every part of the body. You can move a toe under the brain's instructions, and that toe also tells your brain when it has struck something painfully. Significantly, with nerve endings in the bone marrow (the birthplace of white cells), the brain influences the mighty immune system. In addition, your brain is a gland that secretes hormones that affect the entire endocrine system.

Just how deep the mind-body connection is remains somewhat of a mystery; however, every physician knows about the reality of the placebo effect. A placebo is an inert, virtually useless substance (a sugar pill, if you will) sometimes administered to a patient (normally in trials for new medications) under the pretense that it is a powerful drug that will directly improve their condition. Results from the administration of placebos have indeed demonstrated improvement or "healing" in statistically significant numbers of patients. Likewise, upon learning that their "medicine" was not what they believed it to be, some patients have experienced a reversion to their original sickness. There is no explanation for this outside of the influence of thought and feelings on the whole person. You have heard the adage "You are what you eat." You are also what you think.

The implications are so marked that some refer to it as the "biology of belief."[5] This intertwining of influence between body, mind, and spirit has dramatic effects on our overall health. It is in the body with its strengths and weaknesses; the brain/mind with its thoughts, feelings, and consciousness; and the spirit with its committed trust in God and communion with Him that health and wholeness can be ultimately restored to our entire person. It all began with God's intention out of His heart of love to create us in His image to become sons and daughters in Him—forever.

INNER HEALING

It has been observed that hopelessness breeds recklessness— or we might use the term *imbalance*. And to enjoy mental and emotional health, we must have balance that comes through faith impacting our reasoning. This necessary balance for inner health derives from an understanding of and appreciation for the Creator's wisdom. As we cultivate an intimate relationship with God through faith in Christ, we gain appreciation for God's wisdom regarding our lives.

Without that wisdom, people may seek escape from life's difficult challenges and emotional pain through the use of damaging substances and the practice of harmful behaviors. That unhealthy retreat into self-destructive compulsions and addictions is frequently seen as a substitute for the rest and relief that God offers to every person who receives Him in redemption. That kind of false retreat from life's suffering is a grave mistake. Those errant behaviors only complicate things, damage health, and further alienate our hearts from others, our Creator, and our divine purpose.

When you are faced with symptoms of mental or emotional illness, you are presented with something that might very well be life changing in a variety of ways. But in a positive light, through that distress you are afforded the opportunity to contemplate your life and to discover emotional transformation and growth. You will ask, "How can I make sense of what is happening? How can I remain hopeful? How can I live?" when you are weak and the negative emotion of fear becomes your primary sense. These and other questions, when directed to your loving heavenly Father, can bring you to an understanding of His love and purpose for you that can bring healing and wholeness to your inner being.

PERSONALITY

Biology plays a large part in the development of your personality, your mental and emotional perspectives, as do life experiences—whether healthy or harmful—you are exposed to from birth. But you also have choices to make. For example, choosing to live a life of prayer and faith in God has been demonstrated to result in lower levels of inner hostility and higher levels of hope. You and I must learn to appreciate our eternal design and the purposes of our designer for our inner health and wholeness. It is vital that we comprehend the immensity of the impact our hopeful (or hopeless) mentality has on our health. As Dutch Sheets writes, "Hope deferred is the common cold of the soul, except that this virus can kill."[6]

Our Creator endowed us with the inner capacity for hope; it is part of His design for healing. As we wait on God in prayer and believe the promises of His Word for our wholeness, we will nurture that capacity for a hope-filled life. The impact of a hopeful perspective in the process of healing is as powerful as any medication, treatment, or nutrient.

"God meant it for good" (Gen. 50:20). Humans cannot live without hope, without the sense that something good can be attained as we place our trust in God. For example, you must consider that there are many ways the hurtful experiences of your past could result in something good for your future. Your ability to hope in God's love, to express gratitude to God for rescuing you, and to search for God's purpose within that pain is a central key to healing.

CAN HOPE BE AN ESSENTIAL ELEMENT IN THE CURE?

Faith gives substance to hope (Heb. 11:1). Hope is important, but hope lacks substance until it is rooted in faith. I like breaking down the acronym FAITH this way: fully assured I trust Him! Hope is faith talking aloud, drowning out voices of defeat. An example is found in Mark 5, where the woman with the issue of blood expressed her faith, "If only I may touch His clothes, I shall be made well" (v. 28). Hope gave her the tenacity to press forward and declare her faith in Christ. The Amplified Classic Bible says, "For she *kept saying*, If I only touch His garments, I shall be restored to health" (emphasis added).

Hope is birthed in a heart filled with gratitude. You can hope in God because you are assured of His loving character and His promises to hear your cry and answer you (Jer. 33:3; Matt. 7:7). You can develop a habit of expressing thankfulness toward God for His redemption and the love He has shown you. That attitude of gratitude puts you in a frame of mind to expect to receive what you need in His love and what you enjoy in the future He has prepared for you in resting in His redemption. Conversely, an attitude of cynicism and criticism squelches your gratitude to God and hinders your hope and faith in His goodness. These negative mindsets usually are rooted in resentment or bitterness caused by a painful experience for which you have not yet asked forgiveness. Without allowing the Holy Spirit to cleanse you of negative attitudes, you will be hindered in moving forward into a deeper relationship with God and into stronger hope and faith to receive His promises for your life.

Your words are seeds that will bring a harvest. You can express faith and gratitude to God even in your trying situations, and those seeds will bring a harvest of love and life. You can energize others by speaking words of hope and encouragement into their lives in their difficult situations. The Scriptures are clear about the power in our spoken words:

"Death and life are in the power of the tongue" (Prov. 18:21). Regardless of the painful circumstances that created your inner wounds, you can be healed by God's redeeming love as you call on Him and receive His promises to make you whole. As you learn to trust the character of God, you will discover that He never fails.

To share words of hope with an emotionally drowning soul is to drag them into the "life raft" of God. A man or woman whose hope is in the Lord cannot be defeated. To that person, God is always bigger than the giants of their promised land of abundance and wholeness. God desires that our psyche and emotions be restored to rest in His redemption. Embracing the truths in God's Word brings hope for despair, and healing for wounds, no matter what or who caused them. Saturating our souls in His Word enables us to rise above hopelessness and despair.

When the Israelites first arrived at the Promised Land, twelve spies went in to see it. Ten spies returned to the people with an evil report of the giants in the land in whose sight they were like grasshoppers. However, two spies, Caleb and Joshua, brought back a different report. They saw the giants in the land, but they declared their faith in God, knowing that He would help them overcome all the giants to fulfill His promise to them that they would live in the Promised Land.

Joshua and Caleb were filled with hope and faith in God against all the odds they knew were against them. It isn't human nature to hope against hope. In fact, such a response seems contrary to human sanity, but an irrepressible trust in God is always rewarded by fulfilled promises. (See Romans 4:13–25.) And God's peace passes understanding and human reasoning even in the face of challenging situations (Phil. 4:6–7). Joyous faith founded in hope cannot be explained; it is steadfastly based on believing that God will bring the answer to our faith, which is "the substance of things hoped for, the evidence of things not [yet] seen" (Heb. 11:1; see also

1 Pet. 1:7–8). Hope breaks out of the limitation of our mental reasoning and moves forward to receive the promise (the evidence) in faith and confidence in God and His Word.

Hebrews 6:18–19 tells us that when disappointment and confusion come, our response should be to run to the Lord with faith in His power and goodness, not sink into despair. As we remember God's faithfulness in times past, we are enabled to hope again and to share this hope with others. Hope is "an anchor of the soul, both sure and steadfast" (v. 19).

As we receive God's Word into our hearts through faith, hope rises within us. When we live out our faith and hope before others, Paul taught that we become as living "epistles of Christ…written not with ink but by the Spirit of the living God…on tablets of flesh, that is, of the heart" (2 Cor. 3:3). His Word of life transforms us and fills our hearts with faith.

Those who see our witness to Christ receive His life-giving hope as if they were reading the written epistles in the Scriptures. Their faith in Him can be strengthened when they see we are anchored in Him—in His promises by faith! In the troubled times in which we live, Christians whose lives are anchored in the rock, Christ Jesus, and are speaking words of faith and hope will be able to extend a hand of hope to those terrorized by current events. As believers we can learn to say to ourselves:

> Why art thou cast down, O my soul? and why art thou disquieted in me? hope thou in God: for I shall yet praise him for the help of his countenance.
> —PSALM 42:5, KJV

The powerful, living Word of God, applied by the power of the Holy Spirit in the name of Jesus to any situation, quickens the life-changing promises of God. As long as you are content with a thimbleful of God, you will only view life from the standpoint of reports of illness, bad relationship scenarios, and hopeless circumstances, and your soul will be troubled as a result. Determine to cultivate an intimate relationship with God and hope in His Word—and divine power will transform your thinking and make you into a man or woman of faith. The Word of God comes alive in you when you call upon the Holy Spirit of God to awaken your spirit and soul to who God is. Your faith will become like that of Jeremiah, who declared of God: "There is nothing too hard for thee" (Jer. 32:17, KJV).

DISCUSSION ❦ QUESTIONS

Describe a person or situation in your life that brought you hope. Did that hope last or was it temporary?

....

....

....

....

What does hope mean to you?

....

....

....

....

Write a scripture that reminds you of the hope you have in Christ.

....

....

....

....

CHAPTER 3

OBSTACLES TO
INNER HEALING

A S WE HAVE discussed, learning to seek God and rest in the peace, hope, and love of His redemption is the key to inner healing. However, we all experience obstacles to fully entering this divine rest God designed us for and redeemed us to enjoy. These obstacles are largely internal, residing in our minds and hearts as wounds or negative attitudes from which we have not been set free. And they are persistent. These spiritual obstacles damage our well-being, cause us to injure our relationships with others through our reactions to them, and prevent the inner healing and the abundant life that Christ offers. They separate us from total reconciliation to our Creator and Savior and blind us to His eternal plan for our present and future.

UNFORGIVENESS MAKES US ACCUSERS

When a colleague and I suffered great financial loss through unjust trickery, my colleague became miserable because of the anger he harbored against those who had wronged us in a legitimate business transaction. In order for me to escape the same fateful reaction, I knew it was vitally important that I forgive these people and not allow resentment to dwell in my mind and heart against them. I am humbled and deeply grateful for the power of God to keep me resting in His redemption in that unfortunate situation.

In our own strength we cannot maintain the right attitude when we are facing injustice or other difficult situations. We automatically become *accusers* of those who have wronged us unless we make a conscious decision to become an *intercessor* for them. To intercede in prayer for those who have harmed us, to forgive injustice, and to love our enemies as Christ taught us to do (Luke 6:27–36) requires an intimate relationship with our God of love. Only His divine love in our hearts can motivate us to forgive and pray for those who have wronged us. God's forgiving heart will flow into ours as we determine to rest in His grace and redemption.

Apart from that divine grace we receive from our Redeemer, we are doomed to a hellish existence. Our minds and hearts will be filled with strife and ill-at-ease feelings as we face life's challenges. The apostle John shared the desire of God for all believers to have healthy souls and to receive the blessings of God: "Beloved, I wish above all things that thou mayest prosper and be in health, even as thy soul prospereth" (3 John 2, KJV).

Our souls prosper when we cultivate the mystery of divine romance with our Redeemer. When we wait on Him in prayer and in reading His Word, He gives us peace of mind that passes understanding, as I mentioned. He establishes healthy emotional responses in us as we face the most difficult situations of life. Enjoying God and resting in His redemption are eternal gifts that alone can satisfy the human spirit. We are made for Him and destined to glorify Him in all we do. That includes forgiving others when we suffer injustice at their hands.

Jesus taught us to pray, "Forgive us our debts, as we forgive our debtors" (Matt. 6:12). And He taught that it is imperative to forgive our enemies if we are to have fellowship with God. "For if you forgive men their trespasses, your heavenly Father will also forgive you. But if you do not forgive men their trespasses, neither will your Father forgive your trespasses" (vv. 14–15). It is His divine love alone that will empower you to forgive those who have hurt you the most deeply.

Going further, Jesus taught us not only to forgive our enemies, but to "love your enemies, do good to those who hate you, bless those who curse you, and pray for those who spitefully use you." (Luke 6:27–28). Becoming an intercessor for our enemies will be a powerful weapon to cleanse our hearts of the accusation we feel they deserve. God had us in mind when He commanded us to forgive, to love, and to intercede for our enemies.

It is a known scientific fact that resentment, bitterness, and unforgiveness harbored in the mind and heart will cause not only emotional distress but also physical disease as well. Jesus had your well-being in mind when He made it a divine requirement to walk in forgiveness toward others. He wants nothing to hinder you from living in intimate fellowship with Him. He wants nothing to keep you from experiencing the inner healing He has provided for your mind, emotions, and physical being. He is interested in your peace and joy, which are not possible without walking in total forgiveness.

I believe that this strong tendency in us to become *accusers* against our enemies instead of *intercessors* for their souls is one of the greatest hindrances and obstacles to our inner healing. It is one of the greatest causes of inner unhealthiness, which as I mentioned, science has confirmed. We need to change our focus from the wrong done to us and see the wrongdoer through the eyes of God as a sinner who desperately needs God's love and forgiveness. To receive inner healing and become victorious Christians, we must focus our lives on eternal values. Only as we yield our hearts and minds by faith to embrace the truth of God's Word will we enjoy a life of resting in His redemption. As we do, the power of His Holy Spirit working in us will cleanse our hearts from all hatred, bitterness, and resentment as we obey God's Word to forgive our enemies. And we will experience the divine inner healing Christ provided for us in His death at Calvary.

As we discuss other obstacles that hinder your faith for inner healing, I invite you to identify any that might be preventing you from focusing on eternal values that will facilitate health and wholeness in your relationship with God. I encourage you to courageously confront them in faith, believing that God wants you to be healed. By surrendering yourself completely to God in faith, you can overcome any distraction that would keep you from resting in His redemption. The list of these self-deceptions is long and mostly familiar. We will now explore some of these obstacles, which are very significant within the context of our need for inner healing.

Pride

Humility is a godly mindset that is totally aligned with the Creator's design for our inner healing. And there is an enormous hindrance to attaining this godly mindset: pride. What the Bible says about pride's destructive power is extensive and profound. But simply stated, pride prevents us from receiving the whole concept of God's redemption for our entire humanity—body, mind, and spirit.

Pride, more than anything else, blinds us to the physical intricacies of creation and God's special purpose for it. Our scotomas, or blind spots, hide the irreducible complexity, power, and divine wisdom in the design of the human body, psyche, and spirit, which originated with a single, tiny zygote. The pride of man is unwilling to acknowledge God as One to whom we are accountable as the Creator of such complexity. This incontrovertible pride has allowed cold, indifferent, even dubious theories of evolution to gain prominence and influence over generations of minds.

Pride, then, prevents us from acknowledging the majesty of the Creator. Pride refuses to worship Him in awe and appreciation for the magnificence of creation as seen under the microscope and through the telescope. So pride, perhaps more than anything else, separates us from God's grace, His plan, and the eternal meaning and purpose for our lives. It follows that pride is the obstacle that separates us most ably from our inner healing and reconciliation in every aspect of our lives to the majestic Creator and Redeemer of mankind.

The root of pride is selfishness and unwillingness, through fear and arrogance, to surrender to God's sovereignty. Pride is sin that originates within the heart. It may owe its power for some to their undue trust in petty human knowledge and abilities (1 Cor. 8:1). Others develop their scotomas (blind spots) through a sense of self-righteousness, a sense of independence, or the artificial stature encouraged by knowledge, power, and wealth.

Pride will deceive you—blind you—while leading you into relational struggles with others, causing you to develop a spirit toward others that criticizes and injures. Most significantly, pride causes you to reject the Creator and the redeeming truth of His Word. This arrogant mindset amounts to a refusal to see God's handiwork in the marvels of nature and His miraculous design for your life and health. Without worshipful recognition of the divine source of healing, how can you experience it?

Unbridled pride will never result in growth, learning, or healing. Pride can only leave you living in a world of shame, debasement, and destruction. The Scriptures are clear: "When pride comes, then comes shame; but with the humble is wisdom" (Prov. 11:2). And again, "Pride goes before destruction, and a haughty spirit before a fall" (Prov. 16:18). Only your heart, designed and constructed by the Creator to be the seat of your inner man, holds the capacity for genuine understanding. It is there that you yield to the wisdom of humility to give entry to the Creator's plan for your life. His plan is not only temporal but eternal as you receive His divine capacity to love and be loved. You will be astonished at the healing you can experience through your love for God and your fellow man. How you respond to and love others is the measure of your alignment to God.

A critical spirit

At one point in his life E. A. Seamands left his successful career as an engineer to become a missionary in India, extracting his wife from her refined surroundings in the United States and settling in a developing country with a meager one-hundred-dollar-a-month income. The two of them embarked on a mission that lacked not only a piano and a car but even running water and indoor plumbing. Once they were in India, Mrs. Seamands complained loudly and incessantly. Surprisingly, even colleagues suggested to him that he would do well to divorce her.

Mr. Seamands' patient response to this was to say, "I can divorce her as you suggest, but that would not be what the Lord would want me to do. Alternatively, I can separate myself from her and her complaining and continue living the way that I want to live. Or I can constantly pray for her and be an intercessor for her rather than her accuser." He decided to become this intercessor—to assist his wife rather than destroy her.

Through this difficult period Mr. Seamands surmounted the challenges of life and of his relationship with his wife. As he yielded to God in prayer and obedience, he became stronger. As he constantly prayed for his wife, she also became stronger and more tolerant of the life God had ordained for them. Eventually the family ministry flourished through this couple. Mr. Seamands' love for his wife and his effort to align himself with God's higher way (i.e., to intercede for his wife) was the catalyst to set her free from her critical attitudes and constant bickering.

It is too easy to succumb to the temptation of a harboring a critical spirit. Therefore, it is important for you to live above the complaints and criticisms of others. As we discussed, it is necessary to intercede for them rather than accuse them because of their poor attitudes and behavior. Accusations lead nowhere—except to acrimony and conflict. The only possible result of such bitter criticism is division and pain; there is no healing to be found there.

Criticism of another may have a momentary purpose of giving satisfaction if it makes you feel smarter or superior than another. But real purpose is found in your alignment with God's desire that you love, forgive, and appreciate other people. By doing those things, you will find an anointed purpose to your life that will be deeply satisfying. Learning to love, forgive, intercede for, and appreciate others will require that you die to self, that you unite your heart with God's loving heart. Only as you learn to move beyond the obstacle of a critical spirit will you find inner healing for yourself and be able to share that healing power with your loved ones and humanity.

A spirit of envy

One of our most intense inner battles is against a spirit of envy. Few inner states have the same potential to destroy and cause suffering to you and those around you. Envy reflects a selfish desire to have what another possesses, whether relationships, prestige, financial resources, or other things you wish you had. It cloaks itself as a way to pull someone down in the esteem of others, to reduce that person's status because of what you want. Envy is a two-edged sword. While inflicting damage on another, it can rob you of inner health and well-being.

The brutal influence of envy can be seen in the relationships of the world's first family. God smiled on Adam and Eve's son Abel and his offering of a lamb in worship to God. But God was displeased with their son Cain and his offering of vegetables. Cain, consumed by his jealousy of his brother Abel, was overcome with anger and took the opportunity to commit the first murder recorded in the earth. This murderous end of envy is the outcome of allowing selfish desire to fill your heart against another.

A stone is heavy, and the sand weighty; but a fool's wrath is heavier than them both. Wrath is cruel, and anger is outrageous; but who is able to stand before envy?

—PROVERBS 27:3–4, KJV

It is a simple task to prove the repercussions of wrath as a destroyer of hope and loving communication. But envy is described as an abyss, an overwhelming weight before which no one can stand. *Envy* is a four-letter word that personifies the meaning of selfishness. It represents a desire to possess what does not belong to you, as I mentioned. It is insatiable, never to be satisfied until something or someone has been wrecked in the vain pursuit to possess. Once that climax has been enacted, of course, the original object of envy's desire is no longer worth possessing.

As Cain discovered the hard way, nothing is solved by giving in to envy rather than seeking spiritual alignment with God and His peaceful, loving ways. An envious heart is filled with anxiousness and tension begging to be released. That monstrous, sinful attitude results in physical illness, emotional extremes, impaired judgment, and the destruction of the peace and well-being of other people. Such an obstacle removes all possibility for the alignment necessary for the person's inner healing. Envy consumes the energies of body, mind, and heart. The only possible outcome of unmitigated envy is illness, mental breakdown, and spiritual death. The only way out of envy's grip is in realignment with the Lord.

Sadly, if you are already ailing, ill, or in pain, you may become vulnerable to the danger of envying others who do not suffer as you do. It is a small step toward envying others their vitality and physical or mental freedom. The phenomenon is not unusual; however, it demonstrates that part of the process for your inner healing includes the eradication of negative emotions and imaginings. True inner healing that aligns you with the loving heart of the Father can occur only in the absence of envy. Wholeness—freedom from mental and emotional turmoil—can be found as you seek God to forgive you for envy and receive His love that fills your heart.

Independence

When we do not focus our lives on eternal values, it is a sign we are living independently, apart from the love and grace of the Redeemer that brings true inner healing. Independence, which is at the root of all sin, will distract us from fulfilling our God-given purpose. It is our utter dependence on and abandonment to Christ that lead us into God's wonderful redemption rest and healing for body, mind, and spirit. That is what Christ is requiring of us when He asks us to deny ourselves, take up our cross, and follow Him (Matt. 16:24). Denying ourselves is actually a requisite for our inner healing, causing us to abandon ourselves to the eternal love of our God.

Dependence on God means we are resting in Him and acknowledging we can do nothing without Him. Independence means we are living on our own; we have our own agenda. We go our merry way, do our own thing, and leave God and others out of our decisions. Conversely, dependence unites us to God and to the family of God. Acknowledging our need for interdependence lets us relate properly to the body of Christ as His children; independence makes us live as orphans, removed from the loving care of our heavenly Father.

When we commit our lives to the Spirit of God, we acknowledge that we cannot do anything without His love, His grace, or His person. He becomes the consummation of our life. As a result of being totally dependent upon Him, our lives are filled with His peace and joy, and we experience inner healing, resting in His redemption alone. There is no room for the turmoil of selfish desires or negative mindsets that are obstacles to our peace and well-being.

Lack of submission

Closely related to the obstacle of an independent nature is a blatant lack of submission to God's love and purpose for our lives. It is because of our independence that we refuse to submit to the lordship of Christ. Yet experiencing inner healing requires our complete submission to our Lord, which is dependence on Him.

The idea of submission is foreign to most of us; we want to be in control and manage every aspect of our lives. This rebellion against the authority of Christ in our lives results in many difficulties. The Scriptures teach that "the way of the transgressors is hard" (Prov. 13:15, KJV). Yet sometimes, even unwittingly, many in our world today have chosen to walk in their own way without seeking God's blessing for their lives.

Our submission to Christ removes the destructive influences that make our lives so hard. Only as we learn to become truly submissive to the Lord Jesus can we rest in His redemption and be cleansed from the lack of submissiveness in our rebellious hearts. It is beautiful to behold the lives of those who have truly bowed their will to the lordship of Christ. We must bow in submission and servanthood to Christ in order to find the true peace and inner healing He came to give us.

Ingratitude

Ingratitude is the first cousin to discontentment. It is characterized by a terrible lack of appreciation for the blessings we enjoy every day.

The human heart is naturally ungrateful and always covets more than it has unless it submits to the lordship of Christ. In that place of humble submission our eyes will be opened to the wonder of God's supernatural grace working in our lives. As we find true contentment in His love and in communion with Him, He satisfies our hearts with His purposes for our lives and we will become forever grateful.

Becoming radically grateful is a powerful antidote for

most sins we consider "respectable." In truth, there is nothing respectable about sin. Only as we recognize it and ask the Holy Spirit to cleanse us can we be rid of the hindrances sin causes to our inner healing.

Sins we tolerate

Some of the undetected obstacles to our inner healing involve sins we tolerate. These sins are not considered to be a violation of God's laws or love; they are accepted by society. Jerry Bridges has written a book called *Respectable Sins,* which lists many sins some Christians tolerate. Some of these mind-sets have already been discussed, but I felt it was important to share many from his list, since these sins become "hidden" obstacles to our inner healing. As you consider each one, ask the Holy Spirit to show you if any of these are hindering your inner healing and ultimately keeping you from resting in the redemption of God.

- Ungodliness—This is a mindset that is not focused on God or oriented toward Him.

- Anxiety and frustration—Both of these block us from resting in God's redemption.

- Discontentment—This is often over situations that cannot be changed.

- Unthankfulness—This is not being appreciative for all the signs of God's goodness and tokens of His love that are brought into our lives every day.

- Pride—This is being focused on our way or our view, exalting ourselves so we don't rest in Him or surrender to Him so we can rest.

- Selfishness—A selfish life is focused on "me first," always asking, "How does this affect me?

What can I get out of it?" Certainly this is the opposite of resting in His redemption.

- Lack of self-control—This is not being willing to resist the devil and submit to God, or not being willing say no and stand against dead-end roads that hinder us from walking with God.

- Impatience and irritability—These lead in the opposite direction from resting in His redemption. We want things to be convenient and we want things now, instead of resting and waiting on the Lord as Psalm 37:7 teaches.

- Anger—This is certainly an obstacle to inner healing. Something displeases us and we respond with harshness, coldness, and withdrawal. These angry responses show our hearts are not resting in Him. We need to surrender to God, casting our burdens on Him and knowing that pleasing Him is what counts as we declare, "Thy will be done."

- Judgmentalism—These attitudes hinder us from resting in His redemption. Having a critical spirit, fault-finding, nitpicking, and holding unwarranted bias against others certainly reflects a spirit that is not resting in God's redemption.

- Envy and jealousy—These are reflected in not wanting others to have good things or be esteemed because we want those things for ourselves. This uncharitable attitude is a result of not finding our all in our Redeemer and resting in Him as the source of our joy and contentment.

- Worldliness—Even good desires may go beyond their bounds and become obsessive, causing

us to live for the creation and not the Creator,
loving His gifts but denying the Giver.[1]

Unless we identify and repent from these "respectable" sins
that we tolerate in our lives, we will be hindered in our fellowship with Christ and we will not experience the inner healing
we need. Tolerating "respectable" sins, which God does not
tolerate, impedes our communion with Him and hinders any
chance of inner healing we might desire.

DISCUSSION ✿ QUESTIONS

Which of Jerry Bridges' "respectable" sins have you identified in your own life?

....

....

....

....

Is independence or lack of submission a factor that might be preventing your inner healing? Explain.

....

....

....

How does your relationship with Christ provide the source of your happiness, peace, and inner healing?

....

....

....

....

CHAPTER 4

PRESCRIPTION FOR
INNER HEALING

W E HAVE DISCUSSED our need for inner healing of our psyche and emotions, and we have also discussed some of the obstacles in our lives that hinder us from enjoying the peace of God that is our source of inner health. In order for us to receive the inner healing we need, it will be helpful to look more closely at Jesus' divine prescription for our health and wholeness in body, soul, and spirit.

Jesus said to the Pharisees, who were the religious leaders of Israel, "Those who are well have no need of a physician, but those who are sick.... I did not come to call the righteous, but sinners, to repentance" (Matt. 9:12–13). Jesus is telling them clearly that receiving spiritual health requires an acceptance of our need for repentance. The Pharisees did not believe they needed the healing ministrations of the great physician. Therefore, they were incapable of experiencing His healing prescription for the soul because they did not think they needed the heavenly cure.

It is important to put into context the description of the Pharisees of Jesus' day. Bound to fulfilling the law of external religious rituals, many of which had been added to the Law of God, these religious leaders were inflated with a sense of their own righteousness and moral standing in the community. However, their hearts were full of evil contradictions. Jesus taught the people to *observe* the Law of Moses that the Pharisees taught but not to do as the Pharisees did, "for they say and do not do. For they bind heavy burdens, hard to bear, and lay them on men's shoulders; but they themselves will not move them with one of their fingers. But all their works they do to be seen by men" (Matt. 23:3–5).

Earlier we discussed the obstacle of pride that effectively keeps us from receiving the inner healing of God by our refusal to acknowledge Him as our Creator and accept our need for Him to be our Savior. The Pharisees, though religious leaders, suffered from excessive pride and did not humbly acknowledge their need for God. Jesus highlighted their hypocrisy, saying that they were intent on cleaning the outside of the "cup" for appearances, but their hearts were "full of extortion and self-indulgence" (Matt. 23:25).

When we are handed the divine prescription for inner healing as offered to us through Christ, it is in humility that we reach out and take it into our hearts. That posture of humbly recognizing our need of God's cleansing and forgiveness will make His prescription 100 percent effective in making us whole in body, soul, and spirit. As with any medical prescription offered to us by a physician, it can only be effective to bring healing if we take it according to the directions prescribed. In our following discussion, we will look closely at the divine prescription Christ made possible for our inner healing through His death on the cross for our salvation.

Repentance

Why did the Pharisees not see that they needed repentance? What blinded them to their pride, their pompous attitudes and actions, and their mistreatment of their fellow man? Surely their focus on external rules that they touted as "righteousness" played a big part in their deception. And their desire to look good to others while hiding their true motivation did as well.

Each one of us has experienced the sense of guilt for wrongdoing. Do you try to compensate for that guilt with "righteous" external actions for which you believe people will commend you, as the Pharisees did? If so, Jesus offers cleansing of your heart through repentance.

Unlike the Pharisees, you must recognize your need for a physician to cleanse the inner person rather than simply washing the outside of the cup with good outward actions. You must accept His prescription of repentance, which involves turning from your sin to the Savior, in order to receive inner healing. You must ask Him for the forgiveness you need for wrong attitudes and for not acknowledging your need of His righteousness.

All nonbelievers must do these things to accept Christ's forgiveness initially and receive His salvation for their souls. And all believers must ask Christ to cleanse their minds and hearts when they recognize sinful traits—such as resentment, bitterness, and criticism—festering in their hearts. The Son of God must cleanse the dirty, murky waters of our souls. He sends the Holy Spirit to convict and cleanse us of unconscious sin in our heart and to make rivers of living water flow out of our innermost being (John 7:37–39).

Repentance always includes a new obedience to God. The apostle Paul calls us to present all of our members and faculties to be engaged in a life of holiness. (See Romans 6:19.) Peter reminds New Testament believers that what God said of old still applies to us: "Be holy, for I am holy" (1 Pet. 1:16). It is interesting to note that the English words *wholeness* and *holy* derive from the same root. In reference to God the word *holy* means worthy of whole devotion; in believers it speaks of being wholly devoted to God. The original biblical words for *holy* in both Hebrew and Greek mean set apart. They remind us that God is set apart above all

His creation and set apart from sin. For believers it means to be set apart to God as your Lord and your portion in life.

This is why the Bible teaches that true wholeness of our entire being is found only in the measure of holiness we reflect in our relationship with God. True happiness is found in holiness. Spiritual healing is found in holiness. Holiness is ultimately something positive. It is being devoted to God. God's ways for us are designed to meet all of our needs. Behind each command of God's Word are the Father's love and wisdom. Therefore, to seek spiritual healing will always mean realignment with the Word of God—with God Himself—through repentance.

Repentance is never possible without faith in God's Word. Faith is the act of casting ourselves upon Jesus with faith in His promises to give us eternal life. He says, "Come to Me…and I will give you rest" (Matt. 11:28). Faith is acting upon that invitation. The writer of the Book of Hebrews described it as running to Him. Faith is receiving Him as the Bread of Life, our Savior, our Deliverer. Faith is seeking an intimate relationship with God in which we will find all that we need. Faith is learning to enjoy the rest of His redemption in our body, soul, and spirit.

God calls us to find our total satisfaction in Him. Do you see your need of forgiveness because of your sin? The penalty for your sin on the cross is revealed through His suffering. "In Him we have redemption through His blood, the forgiveness of sins, according to the riches of His grace" (Eph. 1:7). Do you need a new heart? He is the One who pours down the Holy Spirit from heaven to change you. Do you need spiritual healing? He is the One who gives the balm of Gilead (Jer. 8:22).

Salvation

The word translated "salvation" in the New Testament is derived from the Greek word *sozo*, defined variously as cure, make well, get well, and restore, as well as save. Salvation through Christ is our divine prescription for healing and health. Two aspects of salvation make it so. First, our salvation was *purchased* for us through Christ's death and resurrection. Second, we must *receive* His salvation through faith.

Our eternal salvation was purchased for us and rests in the imputation of Christ's righteousness to our account, not in our self-righteousness seen in external deeds. Our justification in God's eyes is dependent on Christ's sacrifice for our sins on Calvary: "Therefore, having been justified by faith, we have peace with God through our Lord Jesus Christ, through whom also we have access by faith into this grace in which we stand" (Rom. 5:1–2). Peace with God, our inner wholeness, is possible because of Jesus' work on the cross. He bore the penalty due your sins, and He offered up His perfect life as a sacrifice so that you could receive the righteousness of His obedience. He became our divine prescription for being restored to peace with God and inner wholeness. The Bible is quite emphatic about the foundational truth that our eternal salvation is based on Christ's death:

> …being justified freely by His grace through the redemption that is in Christ Jesus.
> —ROMANS 3:24

> For He made Him who knew no sin to be sin for us, that we might become the righteousness of God in Him.
> —2 CORINTHIANS 5:21

The second aspect of salvation is that we must receive it by faith in a profound way that transforms us to the core of our being. Many profess to believe in Christ with their intellect, but they have not surrendered to Christ through repentance unto salvation. True salvation through faith changes us from a person who is self-centered to one who is God-centered and others-centered. In obedience to God there must be a focus on our caring and compassion for others as well as our passion for God. The two greatest commandments God gave are "love the Lord your God with all your heart" and "love your neighbor as yourself" (Matt. 22:37, 39). True salvation results in a life lived to please God and to care for others. Resting in His redemption is reflected in our obedience to God through discipleship and our caring for others as He does.

Commitment to the process

Salvation, which brings inner healing and wholeness, is a daily, lifelong process more than it is a single event in our lives. From the moment we repent of our sins and turn to Christ for salvation, we are born again into His kingdom. The changes in our life that begin after the new birth must be continually nurtured as we learn to humble ourselves and focus on God's purposes and love for others.

As a new believer you will learn that there is much to do to grow into Christlikeness. There are many areas of the old life that you must relinquish to "put on the new self" in Christ (Eph. 4:24, NIV). Just as physical health will deteriorate in middle age through personal neglect and harmful living habits, so spiritual wholeness and continued inner health require vigilance, diligence, and constant attention.

Every day of your life you will have a daily and desperate need of the heavenly physician to guard the health of your new self. Only as you daily cultivate your intimate relationship with your lovely Lord, waiting on Him in prayer and learning His precepts through the Word of God, can you maintain inner health. You have a present and pressing need of the Spirit's anointing to renew your mind and increase your vitality of spiritual health as you learn His ways.

We often have difficulty with the discipline this process of inner health demands. When we struggle with being able to receive or embrace Christ with our whole heart, it is simply because it is human nature for us to rest in our own resources rather than turn to God. In our human nature, we suffer from blind spots, obstacles, unbelief, hardness of heart, pride, and the continued temptation of distraction, seeking our own satisfaction in earthly pleasures.

However, God has loving ways of humbling us to bring us to the place where we have nothing else to hold on to but Him. He will make it plain, sometimes through life's difficult circumstances, that we cannot enjoy His provision for resting in His redemption without making our relationship with Him our priority. It is necessary to realize that illness and trials sometimes accomplish this humbling in our lives and that inner healing as well as physical healing occurs when we turn wholeheartedly to God and return to rest in His redemption.

It is in your trials—even of illness—that you may draw closer to Jesus. Joni Eareckson Tada's life is a glowing testimony to this divine reality. She has lived life as a quadriplegic confined to a wheelchair since a terrible diving accident in 1967. Though the radical changes in her life were painful to accept, in that initial bleakness Joni asked God to show her how to live. In the years since her accident Joni has accomplished much. She is a painter, public speaker, author, disability advocate, columnist, and wife. It was through her immense challenges that Joni sought to live closer to her Savior within His plan for her. She knows that by putting one's trust in Christ, concerns of the body become a lower priority. As she writes, "Life is intricately and intimately linked with Jesus. In fact, Jesus is life— He says so Himself. So when we look for life worth living, we must look for it not in happy or heartbreaking circumstances, health, or even relationships. Life is in Christ."[1]

During our times of ease and abundance, we tend to lapse into a feeling of independence and strength in ourselves. However, when life becomes difficult, it presses us up against Jesus. In hard times, in times of crisis, brokenness, and suffering, we learn to depend upon God and His plan. This is healing.

"'Is not My word like a fire?' says the LORD, 'and like a hammer that breaks the rock in pieces?'" (Jer. 23:29). God sends His Spirit and His Word to be a hammer and a fire to break down our inner obstacles and restore us to faith. The soul's malady is purged by these heavenly processes. Yet God uses them to draw us to Himself by the sweetness of His promises wrapped up in the Lord Jesus: "All the promises of God in Him are Yes, and in Him Amen, to the glory of God through us" (2 Cor. 1:20).

Prayer

Answers to prayer bring glory to God because they are the Lord's hand intervening for us. Scientists have found the effects of prayer to have real life confirmations in medical practice.

The most widely cited study to date on the therapeutic effects of prayer was conducted by Dr. Randolph Byrd at the San Francisco Medical Center in 1988. Dr. Byrd studied a coronary care unit (CCU) population to explore two questions:

1. Does intercessory prayer to the Judeo-Christian God have any effect on the patient's medical condition and recovery while in the hospital?

2. How are these effects characterized, if present?[2]

In this study 393 patients were assigned randomly to one of two groups. Group 1 had prayers made to God on behalf of the patients by intercessors associated with study. Group 2, the control group, received no prayers from anyone associated with the study. Intercessory prayer for each member in the first group was exercised by three to seven intercessors who were provided with the patient's first name, diagnosis, and general condition. Intercessors selected were born-again Christians with active Christian lives in their churches. All 393 patients received the same high-quality cardiac care at the hospital. The identities of the individuals in each group were kept secret from the attending doctors, the nurses, and the patients themselves.

Dr. Byrd recorded the dramatic results of his statistical study about the efficacy of remote intercessory prayer.

> Analysis of events after entry into the study showed the prayer group had less congestive heart failure, required less diuretic and antibiotic therapy, had fewer episodes of pneumonia, had fewer cardiac arrests, and were less frequently intubated and ventilated.[3]

Dr. Byrd concluded that with intercessory prayer to God—from a distance and without the beneficiary's knowledge—"there seemed to be an effect, and that effect was presumed to be beneficial."[4]

The apostle Paul taught believers to make prayer a continual conduit of thanksgiving, worship, and petition in daily life. He actually admonished us to "pray without ceasing" (1 Thess. 5:17). How is this possible? It is a little like how often you think about someone when you are in love. There is probably not a waking moment when that person is not on your mind. Our intimate relationship with Christ should be like that as we acknowledge Him in all our ways and give thanks for all the blessings He gives to us daily. When you wake up at night, think of His love for you and not of the world and its anxieties. Be constantly thinking about your Redeemer and about your relationship to Him as you go through your days. Staying in close contact with God will help you when the rough spots in your life occur. He is just a call away.

> Call to Me, and I will answer you, and show you great and mighty things, which you do not know.
> —JEREMIAH 33:3

What I call "breath prayers" have become a true blessing and a refreshing way to "pray without ceasing" as we go through the busy workday at St. Luke's Cataract and Laser Institute. Breath prayers are short, simple requests that can be spoken to God in one breath. They can be a sincere phrase of praise, gratitude, or worship. They can be a petition for one who is facing a difficult situation. Try your own breath prayers—they will keep you focused on your need for and gratitude to God and help you to cope with whatever situations arise in your day. They certainly will remind you of God's continual presence and grace in your daily life. After all, it is His very breath that you are breathing and that gives and sustains your life.

Here are some suggestions for breath prayers you can whisper to God daily:

- Give me gentleness, Father.

- Bring healing to this patient, Father; guide me in my part.

- Bless my children, their spouses, and my grandchildren today, Father.

- Help me better understand and live Your truth today.

- May I live for the anointing, Father; it's the presence of the Holy One.

For a few years our friend Ralph McIntosh battled an aggravating bout of symptoms, including chest pain, which the doctors couldn't define well enough to determine the right treatment. At one point he was hospitalized and tests were run, but still there was no conclusive evidence. A resulting weakness drained his strength so much that he had trouble climbing stairs without pulling himself up one step at a time by clinging onto the handrails. He knew something was terribly wrong with him, but no test pinpointed the problem.

One day while his wife, Susan, was at work, in desperation he determined to seek the Lord's healing for himself. He pulled two chairs together in their living room and sat down to pray, picturing the Lord in the other chair. He spoke aloud, "Jesus, am I dying? If so, I want to know so I can get things in order for my wife and family." For some time he sat there waiting for an answer. Then he sensed that he was in the very presence of the Lord Jesus, communing with Him person to person. He experienced an amazing spiritual moment with the Lord, and from that day forward he began to get well. The weakness left, and his health returned. With that remarkable healing came a renewed purpose and call upon his life. That day, he received not only an inner healing but a spiritual commissioning. Within a few years he gave up his contracting business, and he and his wife went into full-time Christian ministry.

Isaiah had a powerful encounter with God recorded in Isaiah chapter 6. He saw a vision of heaven and realized he was a sinful man. As he acknowledged his need for deeper cleansing, he experienced a heavenly coal of fire laid on his lips. Then he heard a voice say, "Who will go for Us?" And Isaiah's immediate response was, "Here am I! Send me" (v. 8).

Our response to God's glorious presence in those special moments when we sense His nearness will always be to worship Him. And the love His presence evokes in our hearts, followed by a deeper awareness of our need for redemption, will inevitably lead to a new commissioning by God to tell others of His love. With grateful hearts we will say with Isaiah, "Here am I! Send me."

Fellowship

John Donne, a renowned late sixteenth-century English poet and cleric in the Church of England, declared the fundamental truth that "no man is an island" unto himself.[5] Modern social sciences have well-documented evidence that vibrant social bonds are an essential element for health, healing, and longevity.[6] Experience through centuries of studying mankind as a social being has proven the validity of those truths. At St. Luke's we are keenly aware of the beneficial effects that accompany reaching out to the individual patient in a helpful, human, loving manner.

God had good reasons for commanding us to live in unity and in loving fellowship with one another. He established the church to be a safe place, a "body" of believers, as Paul describes it, where all the "joints and ligaments" are needed for the health of Christ's church (Eph. 4:16; Col 2:19). There is something about having to rub elbows with other people that helps us stay involved in lives other than our own. Caring people will notice our emotional struggles and help keep us from isolating ourselves by listening and offering prayer and kindness.

Even family members seem more isolated from each other today, with separate bedrooms for each child, TVs in every room, and involvement in games and personal interests taking the place of real interaction between parents and children and between siblings.

Whether it's a church family, a social club, a gym, a service club, a volunteer position at a hospital, a book club, or a Christian twelve-step support group, relationships provide the opportunity for meeting social and emotional needs by staying in touch with others. Some of the loneliest people wait for their phones or doorbells to ring and complain because no one cares. While that may be an accurate perception for some, we must realize that it is our responsibility to reach out to others as well. More than a responsibility, it is actually a privilege and a basic element for inner health to be involved in others' lives. Even if you aren't a "group" kind of person, you were created to communicate and share life with others, and that is neglected at risk to your inner health.

Medical professionals have evidence that loneliness kills;

we should avoid it like the plague. Psychiatrists at McGill University took a group of heart attack survivors who were being discharged from the hospital and divided them up into two groups. Both groups received the same excellent heart care from the cardiologists and their own family physicians. However, one group also received monthly phone calls from the research team.

If the researcher making the phone contact sensed any psychosocial problem, a specially trained nurse was scheduled to visit the patient in the home. Just the little personal contact made with patients resulted in a 50 percent reduction in the patients' death rate after one year for those who were in the group cared for by occasional phone calls and visits.[7]

All of us need to have meaningful interaction with others in order to enjoy inner health. Our intimate relationship with God enlarges our capacity to reach out to others with His love. That interaction not only encourages and strengthens the person who receives it, but also the person who gives it is refreshed and strengthened as well. It causes us to forget about ourselves when we focus on others. God made us to need one another. We need listening ears and caring hearts, and it must be a two-way street in order for a family, a community, or a church to be made up of healthy, emotionally fulfilled people.

The Scriptures admonish believers to encourage others, pray for others, sing together, and testify of what God is doing in their lives in order to edify—build up—others in Christian love. Your life is enriched when you reach out to others and let them reach out to you. We do live in a fallen world where sin and pain abound. Many times, through no fault of our own, we are victims of wounded hearts because of a relationship gone wrong. Often our tendency is to pull in to ourselves and avoid close relationships to avoid being hurt again. Or sometimes we fear, "If people know this or that about me, they wouldn't want to be my friend."

Those are signs of inner unhealth that need to be brought

to God in prayer for healing, allowing the Holy Spirit to show us the pathway to freedom from those and other negative responses to others. Fellowship with others is a freeing experience. God has placed distinct gifts and aspects of His divine nature within you and within every believer. When you fellowship with others, you can edify others with the beauty of God in your life. We are simply incomplete apart from cultivating fellowship relationships with the other members of the body of Christ.

THE BEATITUDES: A BLESSED MINDSET

Alignment—the term we use to refer to the rest that brings inner healing—really involves abandonment of our lives to God; it means allowing the Holy Spirit to reign within our hearts and minds in all our decisions and every aspect of life. The Lord created us in a wonderful way as complex persons. However, without yielding our lives to His plan for our wonderful redemption, ungodly, destructive, and negative thoughts keep us bound to fear and misery. And we forfeit the wonderful freedom the Holy Spirit desires to give to us.

In developing God's blessed mindset, you take your first step toward true alignment with His design and desire for you. As you cultivate an intimate relationship with Christ, allowing His Word to teach you and to cleanse you of wrong attitudes and thinking patterns, you are on His divine pathway to inner healing. Allowing the work of the Holy Spirit to align your will, mind, and emotions with God's loving redemptive plan for you allows you to experience His blessed mindset and enjoy His consequent inner healing that every soul craves.

The godly attitudes that produce mental health are aligned with the Creator's design for mankind. They are outlined most explicitly in what we refer to as the Beatitudes, found in Matthew 5:3–12. These foundational principles present what is probably the best summary of the blessed mindset of God, which results in inner wholeness. God's blessed mindset produces a life that stands in direct opposition to the life produced by our natural mindset when living under a burden of sin.

The first beatitude says, "Blessed are the poor in spirit, for theirs is the kingdom of heaven" (v. 3). Humility is listed as the first requirement for God's Spirit to transform us. However, we are often preoccupied with self-centeredness and pride. In that ungodly mindset, we are concerned with satisfying what we feel are our needs. How am I going to be hurt? What does that person think about me? How does this make me look? What do I get out of this? The mindset described in the Beatitudes is one that is centered on God and others—not on self. It is a spirit of humility and a focus that is Godward.

The theme of humility continues in the second beatitude, which pronounces God's blessing on the brokenhearted: "Blessed are those who mourn, for they shall be comforted" (v. 4). Matthew is describing people who know the glory of repentance and forgiveness, as David expressed in his prayer in Psalm 51. The Savior told us we are blessed when we mourn over our sin because we will be comforted by God Himself. We can also expect to be comforted in times of mourning caused by life's difficult situations. Life is temporal. Because of the evil influence of our enemy, Satan, it involves suffering. But our growing relationship with the triune God is eternal—promising us life forever in the bliss of His presence.

When our focus is eternal, our earthly suffering pales in that hope. And our loving Savior heals the pain of our hearts as we cultivate our relationship with Him. He promised to send us the Comforter, the Holy Spirit, to strengthen us and comfort our hearts. No matter the devastating earthly circumstances we may face, God's authentic healing touch is eternal and ever present.

"Blessed are the meek, for they shall inherit the earth" (v. 5). *Meekness* is defined as controlled strength. Without the revelation of and obedience to what the Lord would have us accomplish, we would be dangerous. Our natural mind can sometimes tell us to drive to success, disregarding our health or consideration for others, or to exact justice we feel we deserve through our own power. Meekness, however, means living under another's authority—God's authority. Only as we live in obedience to His commands can true justice or success be found. Pride, a true opposite mindset from meekness, will destroy us. In our pride, living independently of God, we cannot inherit His portion for us in this life or in the new heavens and the new earth in eternity.

"Blessed are those who hunger and thirst for righteousness, for they shall be filled" (v. 6). Individuals who reach this fourth beatitude attitude in their pursuit of God's ways are pronounced happy and filled! A basic human flaw affecting every person is that we are full of and bound by selfish desires. Those desires are like thorns that choke the Word of God in our lives. The empty quest to fulfill earthly desires inevitably remains unsatisfied, merely increasing the longing of earthly desires; those desires can never be quenched. It is only as we truly hunger and thirst after God's ways that we will find true heart satisfaction.

The fifth beatitude tells us, "Blessed are the merciful, for they shall obtain mercy" (v. 7). No one is closer to the very heart of Christ Himself than a merciful, forgiving man or woman who is patient with the failures and shortcomings of others. The pathway to one's own inner healing leads to a mindset of nurturing and assisting the healing of others. A merciful heart lacks traces of bitterness, envy, and other negative attitudes. It is distinguished by an unwillingness to hold grudges or aggravate injury. Rather, a merciful mindset empowers you to become an intercessor rather than an accuser, as we discussed earlier. Such a happy soul is God's channel of grace in a world full of hate.

The sixth beatitude is "Blessed are the pure in heart, for they shall see God" (v. 8). This promise is a profound source of encouragement that will keep you moving toward alignment with God, especially during times when you are tempted to go your own way. The wonder of gazing at God's joyful countenance will focus your attention on keeping your heart pure. If you do not keep your eyes on God, you be focused on those things that will ultimately defile you.

The devil's temptations always present you with a beautiful apple without showing you the worm hidden inside that will destroy you. Many peaceful homes and marriages have been ruined by a wandering eye that was diverted from pursuing God. Searching for—and seeing—the face of God, especially during times of temptation, brings release from the temptation and brings spiritual pleasures that are infinitely more satisfying than what the temptation offered.

Peacemakers receive a happy benediction in the seventh beatitude: "Blessed are the peacemakers, for they shall be called sons of God" (v. 9). God's inner healing is found in embracing the gospel—the good news—of the power of reconciliation. People who have become angry and embittered become soft and tender toward one another when yielding to God's powerful blessing of peacemaking. Such sweet fellowship is wonderful evidence that God can change a very powerful negative bent of a soul. Being willing to make peace through forgiveness and reconciliation is a necessity to experience God's inner healing and peace. What a blessing it is to be what Paul calls "God's coworkers" (1 Cor. 3:9, TLB) as we seek to unite others who suffer from hard and bitter hearts.

The final beatitude of blessing is pronounced especially for those who are persecuted for the sake of righteousness. "Blessed are those who are persecuted for righteousness' sake, for theirs is the kingdom of heaven" (Matt. 5:10). One of the heaviest weights for the human spirit to bear is to be falsely accused for good we have done. It is human nature to immediately defend our honor when challenged. In our self-defense we conveniently forget the many times when we were wrong, yet our wrongdoing was neither caught nor exposed. Such selective sight and memory cause us to defend ourselves with great energy and without mercy.

However, to humbly bear the pain of false accusation is to follow the Savior's example. We may be hated, persecuted, or hurt by others' accusations for doing what is right in God's eyes. Jesus tells us to rejoice and be exceedingly glad when that happens because He will reward us greatly in heaven (vv. 11–12). And He will comfort us by the Holy Spirit in our hurtful, unjust situation.

This divine comfort is the foundational promise of all the Beatitudes. As you seek to please God and rest in His redemption, you live contently, knowing that you love your God and aim to please Him. This is the blessed mindset of a life aligned with God. This spiritual alignment with God's loving ways frees you from the destructive thought patterns that ruin your life and relationships and distance you from your Savior. In this blessed alignment you can experience a mindset free to enjoy the liberty that God designed the soul to experience.

DISCUSSION 🌿 QUESTIONS

Has your faith ever had a positive impact on your physical health? Your mental health? Explain.

What painful mental, emotional, or physical symptoms are you experiencing that might be eliminated by pursuing realignment of your life with God's Word and His promises for peace and rest?

What is the first step you will take toward the realignment of your life with God that promises inner healing?

CHAPTER 5

THE ROLE OF FAITH
IN INNER HEALING

WHILE THROUGHOUT THESE pages we have discussed the necessity and power of personal faith in God to make our inner healing possible, I want to focus specifically on how faith works to transform a person—body, soul, and spirit. Even medical science has had to recognize the power of religious faith to effect positive change in a person's health.

Clinical evidence and formal studies have been conducted that prove the positive influence of religious faith on healing. This includes the positive effects of private devotional activities such as the daily reading of God's Word and personal prayer as well as intercessory prayer (praying for others). It also includes fellowship and worship with other believers as part of a local church. These lifestyle practices of believers are so positive that health practitioners are finding the influence of religious faith difficult to ignore.[1] These research studies have been published in a variety of medical journals.[2] For example, studies report the following potential benefits for people who do attend church or profess a faith in God:

- They have a lower risk of heart disease,

- They have improved immune function.

- They have a lower risk of cancer.

- They live longer.[3]

Many people come to know God when suffering unbearable grief, sorrow, or other kinds of trouble for which there is no relief or human solution. As they seek God, they find the comfort and wisdom in His presence they need to give them strength to carry on in life.

Some come to know God through the witness of loving friends or family, whose caring hearts they desire to emulate. When they discover that the source of their friends' love is the love of God, they are inspired to seek God for themselves. Everyone who has surrendered to God has a testimony of how God lovingly drew his or her heart to Himself. Indeed, the Holy Spirit is always working through many different avenues to reveal the love of Jesus to needy, hurting hearts. Churches that preach the true gospel of God's redeeming power; ministers who share the love of God through His Son, Jesus Christ; and believers who allow the love of God to flow through them to others are powerful ways to win lost souls to Christ's love and wondrous redemption.

KNOWING CHRIST VS. KNOWING *ABOUT* HIM

There is a great difference between knowing *about* Christ and truly pursuing intimate relationship with Him as Savior and Lord. Jesus declared: "I am the way, the truth, and the life" (John 14:6). He taught that by believing in Him, we will find true life and the divine rest and peace He came to give to those who receive His salvation by faith. Faith, that deeply personal spiritual conviction, is the key to receiving the atonement of Christ and learning to live in intimate relationship with Him.

It is not knowledge but personal spiritual conviction (faith) that motivates us first to come to Christ. That conviction comes to us through the work of the Holy Spirit who reveals to us the love of Christ and our own sinful ways. It is also that personal conviction that motivates us to follow Him as the *way*, to learn of Him as the *truth*, and to live in Him who is *life*. (See John 14:6.) This personal, living, eternal relationship is much more profound than a mental religious assent to doctrines of the church. In short, knowing Christ intimately through faith transcends the superficial idea of knowing about Him.

The good news is that God gives to each of us "a measure of faith," which empowers us to truly know Christ (Rom. 12:3). According to the Scriptures, salvation is a "free gift" (Rom. 5:16). The apostle Paul explains, "For the wages of sin is death; but the *gift of God* is eternal life through Christ Jesus our Lord" (Rom. 6:23, emphasis added). That wonderful gift of redemption from sin is available to all who will call on the name of the Lord (Acts 2:21). Through the power of the Holy Spirit, we can be born again into the kingdom of God, knowing Christ as our Savior who takes away our sin. That wonderful reality makes the mystery of divine romance with our Creator/Savior available to all who simply ask.

Jesus taught that eternal life means knowing the one true God (John 17:3). Imagine entering into that divine relationship of eternal life while still living on this troubled, chaotic earth. That is what Christ made available to us as we pursue relationship with Him as our Redeemer through faith. Such deep personal conviction lays hold of this spiritual reality and transforms our lives day by day. Walking through life with the divine presence of God directing, protecting, and loving us becomes our eternal focus.

Faith to receive Christ is a gift of God. He calls everyone to believe in Him and to truly know Him. God's love transcends every excuse and fear that people have regarding the gift of redemption through Christ. The greatest moment in the life of any person is when they humble themselves to come to Christ and ask for His forgiveness. From that moment on they are able to begin to live as they were meant to live, justified by faith in God's eyes and receiving His peace (Rom. 5:1).

FAITH THAT CHANGES THE WORLD

As we respond to Christ's invitation to follow Him in genuine faith, based on deep spiritual conviction, our faith will not be diminished by challenging circumstances in the world in which we live. On the contrary, our faith in Christ will help us to change the world, making an impact on others to bring them to Christ. As you cultivate a covenant relationship with your Savior, He will show you how to be effectively involved in meaningful life pursuits.

He will give you wisdom to impact your family, have influence in your career, and be involved in many other worthwhile endeavors to promote the kingdom of God in the earth. When you choose to pursue intimate relationship with your Redeemer, you will learn to rest in His redemption above all else. And life's involvements will become prioritized around this wonderful mystery of divine romance you enjoy with your Lord.

Legitimate, God-given pursuits will become more effective as you mature in your covenant love relationship with your Lord. The more love you receive from Him, the more you will desire to return that love in worship to Him and in fruitful service to others. And your faith will lift and expand the capacity of your heart so that you will lay aside otherwise harmless pursuits that do not contribute to your God-given purpose. Your focus will become eternal rather than temporal, to fulfill those purposes of God in the earth.

The apostle Paul uses the analogy of marriage to describe a believer's relationship to Christ. He tells husbands to love their wives "just as Christ also loved the church and gave Himself for her" (Eph. 5:25). He declares that Christ cherishes the church. To *cherish* (*thalpō* in the Greek) means "to cherish with tender love, to foster with tender care."[4] That humble caring is a description of what covenant love should be between a man and woman in marriage.

Then Paul explains that as believers we are united to Christ in a similar way. He also describes this divine mystery of covenant relationship in terms of our becoming "members of His body, of His flesh and of His bones" (Eph. 5:30). That description does not denote a casual, intellectual relationship with our Lord. It is a spiritual relationship involving personal commitment by the two parties involved. And it results in deep, satisfying intimacy of heart and mind that encompasses every issue of life.

Truly knowing our Creator-Redeemer means our entire being is consummated in His love, in that mystery of divine romance. In spite of our many imperfections we have been united with Christ, who is divine perfection. In our poverty we have been made partakers of the divine riches our Savior provides for us.

To illustrate this wondrous transformation of our lives in Christ, consider the story of a poor country girl who marries a well-to-do, educated, sophisticated young man. They are deeply in love, united with a common respect for each other and for their goals for life. But one partner brings much more "wealth" to the relationship than the other. Immediately after they are married, this girl who was raised in poverty becomes the owner of a beautiful home, drives an expensive car, and enjoys financial security she has never known.

She never forgets the pain of the poverty from which she was rescued, but she cherishes the one who rescued her. That is a picture of the security we have when we abandon ourselves to Christ. He leads us into resting in His redemption by faith and enjoying the wealth of His supernatural lifestyle. The apostle Paul referred to this as "Christ in you, the hope of glory" (Col. 1:27).

Through abandoning ourselves in faith to Christ and living in covenant relationship with Him, we inherit the inner healing, health, and wholeness He has provided for us. It is very important that we not just enter into a "dating" relationship with Christ, flirting with His promises without making a complete commitment of our lives. As we submit our lives to God, our faith will bring us into God's rest: "For we who have believed do enter that rest" (Heb. 4:3). When we enter His rest, we cease from our own works, as God did from His (v. 10). When we allow Christ to become our righteousness, we learn to enjoy His spiritual rest in all of life.

Our priority as believers is to "be zealous and exert ourselves and strive diligently to enter that rest [of God, to know and experience it for ourselves], that no one may fall or perish by the same kind of unbelief and disobedience [into which those in the wilderness fell]" (v. 11, AMPC). Faith—deep personal conviction—is the key to living fruitful lives and enjoying the fulfillment of God's promises for wholeness in our lives. When some asked Jesus how to do the works of God, Jesus declared:

> This is the work of God, that you believe in Him whom He sent.
>
> —JOHN 6:29

Have you considered *believing God* to be your supreme life work? What about believing the wonderful promises of God and entering into the divine romance of walking with the Savior? What about resting in His redemption? The more we commune with God, the closer we come to the purpose for which we were created: to glorify God in all we do and enjoy Him forever.

FAITH AND WORKS

When we pursue an intimate relationship with God by faith according to His Word, we will inevitably seek to express our gratitude by serving others to bring glory to God. The Scriptures show us how to fulfill the real purpose of God for our lives.

> Be renewed in the spirit of your mind, and...put on
> the new man which was created according to God, in
> true righteousness and holiness.
>
> —EPHESIANS 4:23–24

"Without faith it is impossible to please [God]" (Heb. 11:6). As we enter into the rest of His redemption, we will believe His promises through faith. It is clear throughout Scripture that our primary goal in life must be to seek God in faith, to know Him, and to abandon our lives to the mystery of that divine romance.

As we learn to abide in Christ, everything we do will be guided by our passionate love to fulfill the purpose of God in our lives. As we cultivate this intimate relationship with Christ, we hear His voice or are led by the Spirit of God. Our focus must first be on abiding in Him, and then He will lead us into the good works He has ordained for us to walk in (Eph. 2:8–10).

Even when we know we are doing the work God has given us to do, we must continue to focus on our relationship with Him. Otherwise we will find ourselves so consumed with the work of the Lord that we neglect of the Lord of the work. That is a recipe for disaster. Mother Teresa observed,

> There is always the danger that we may just do the
> work for the sake of the work....This is where the
> respect and love and the devotion come in, that we
> give it and do it to God, to Christ and that is why we
> try to do it as beautifully as possible.[5]

She also said,

> Many people mistake our work for our vocation. Our
> vocation is the love of Jesus.[6]

"Our vocation is the love of Jesus." I have been guilty of losing that focus at times in pursuing my personal vocation. Have you? I have become so busy with my medical practice and other responsibilities of family, church, and so on that I forfeit even physical rest. When I was an intern, there were many times when I had very little sleep for days. Even when I tried to sleep, I was unable to rest because I was so "tuned out" to resting.

We miss so much of life as our Lord intended it when we allow our life activities and involvements to spiral out of control. Not only do our bodies suffer, but we also lose the sense of God's presence in our lives when we fail to enjoy the rest for our souls that He offers us. I have learned that the heavier my workload—the greater the stress of demands on my time and energies—the more I need to turn off my worries and totally rest in His redemption.

As I consciously focus on my relationship with Christ and His promises to be there for me, I have found that things get better. I rely on His strength in me to accomplish the tasks at hand. Instead of working harder, I concentrate more on resting in and leaning on Him. Jesus promised that if we would simply come to Him, we would find rest for our souls (Matt. 11:28).

John Wesley, founder of the Methodist Church, reportedly said: "I have so much to do that I spend several hours in prayer before I am able to do it."[7] I had a mentor who used to say that he would pray longer on the days that he had more work to do. Instead of getting up earlier and working longer, he would pray longer. He knew he could not do anything without Jesus. So he began his prayer time by thanking God for planning all of creation and expressing gratitude for Christ's incarnation, becoming man and providing our redemption. He thanked Him for imputing His righteousness to us and making possible the consummation of our love for Him. He could feel his mind relax and his perspective change when he focused in this way on his relationship with God. And he would walk through his day in the strength of the Lord.

The essence of Christianity is that we learn to rest in His grace, His love, His person, and His redemption by faith. To live in that reality, we must learn not to rest in our own accomplishments, abilities, or intellectual conclusions about life. Instead, we focus on the One who cares for our eternal souls and has provided all we need to live victoriously.

Then when challenges, injustices, hurts, and trials come, we know the source of our life. We can turn to Him for wisdom, comfort, grace to forgive, and the ability to love others the way He loves us. That is the benefit of living every moment in dependence on our Redeemer.

LISTEN TO YOUR WORDS

To know if your faith in Christ is leading you into obedience to His kingdom purpose, listen to your words. What are you speaking? Are you focused on your own misgivings, fears, and worries? Your personal success? Are you speaking doubt and worry words? Or are your words filled with faith in His goodness and His eternal care for you?

What are you listening to? Are you receiving false or humanistic teaching that denies the supernatural dimension of a relationship with Christ? Or is your priority to embrace the promises of the Word of God and speak to yourself its truths? The apostle Paul admonishes us:

> Wherefore be ye not unwise, but understanding what the will of the Lord is. And be not drunk with wine, wherein is excess; but be filled with the Spirit; speaking to yourselves in psalms and hymns and spiritual songs, singing and making melody in your heart to the Lord; giving thanks always for all things unto God and the Father in the name of our Lord Jesus Christ.
>
> —EPHESIANS 5:17–20, KJV

The Scriptures have much to say about the power of our words. Paul taught that we must not listen to everything that is spoken, even in the name of church tradition, but that "speaking the truth in love," we will grow into mature Christians (Eph. 4:15). He said we must put off our former kinds of conversation, which were corrupt. Instead, we must "be renewed in the spirit of [our] mind" (Eph. 4:23). Listening to, speaking, and believing the Word of God will restore the peace and joy to our souls that Christ's redemption provides. It is a conduit for our inner healing.

Until we abandon ourselves by faith to the mystery of divine romance with our Savior, we will not fulfill the purpose of the Scriptures for our lives. We will be condemned to living in wearisome self-effort, following rules and gritting our teeth to live peaceably with others. It is the mystery of a love relationship with Christ that sets me free to rest in His redemption. He flows His divine love through my mind and heart for every situation.

Established by faith in Him, I am protected from the peril of unbelief and led into divine purpose for my life. And as I listen to His redemptive Word, I speak in faith what He gives me to speak.

DISCOVERING PURPOSE FOR LIFE

After salvation we learn why we were created anew: to be God's masterpieces, redeemed so we can fulfill the purpose for us that He planned a long time ago. What an incredible thought! The yearning I have to live a purposeful life was put into my heart by God Himself! And it is in abandoning myself to His gift of redemption by faith that I will discover the good things He purposed for me to do. Those purposes will satisfy that yearning of my heart to enjoy God and glorify Him in all I do.

The human soul longs to know that there is a purpose for its existence. The futility of living life with no sense of purpose leads many into despair. In pursuing the mystery of romance with Christ, we learn that God has ordained us for a divine purpose, and He gives us grace to fulfill it. In Christ, every divine hunger of the human heart is realized and inner healing takes place.

Earthly achievements will never replace the need for faith that embraces the truth that God "is a rewarder of those who diligently seek Him" (Heb. 11:6). Personal accomplishments can never fulfill the hunger of the human heart for rest found only in the redemption of Christ. They can never prepare the eternal human soul to live forever with the Creator-Redeemer.

FAITH IS "STANDING"

Faith, defined as our deep personal conviction, stands on the promises of God and determines to walk in the purposes of God regardless of circumstances. You stand on your faith just as you stand on His redemption and His promises. As you focus on the greatness of His redemption, your priority in life is transformed. You do not live to please yourself or to gain personal recognition. You consider Jesus alone in everything you do. By faith you live to please the Lord and to bring glory to His name (Col. 3:17). No challenge is too great for genuine faith:

> Therefore, my beloved brethren, be steadfast, immovable, always abounding in the work of the Lord, knowing that your labor is not in vain in the Lord.
> —1 CORINTHIANS 15:58

As a born-again child of God, learning to walk in His purposes is a result of resting in the redemption of Christ. Fulfilling your divine destiny involves your complete abandonment in faith to intimate relationship with Him. That love relationship is a divine mystery of covenant commitment filled with joy, peace, and contentment. It is the key to freedom from fear and worry.

Learning to abide in Christ enables you to do everything you were meant to do in dependence upon His person. When you make this divine relationship the priority of your life, you will experience true inner healing and be enlarged in your heart and mind to accomplish more than you ever dreamed possible.

DISCUSSION ✿ QUESTIONS

Describe inner healing in your own words.

....

....

....

We receive Christ's redemption when we are justified by faith. Does that result in peace? Can we live in peace without resting in His redemption? Explain.

....

....

....

Is inner turmoil the opposite of resting in His redemption? How does a lack of peace affect your relationship with God, yourself, and others?

....

....

When we enter His rest, do we really cease from our own striving and find true inner healing? Why or why not?

....

....

CHAPTER 6

THE HEALING POWER
OF FORGIVENESS

NNER HEALING—MENTAL, EMOTIONAL, spiritual—will not be fully complete until you have released the last remnant of unforgiveness harbored in your heart against another. Until you truly accept God's forgiveness for your sins and then choose to forgive those who trespass against you, you cannot live in the wholeness God offers you to the fullest degree possible. Unforgiveness, as we discussed, is one of the primary obstacles to your health, especially to your inner healing. Living a life of continual forgiveness for suffered wrongs is one of the key exercises of our hearts and minds in order for inner healing to be our portion.

R. T. Kendall's book *Total Forgiveness* provides us a definitive handbook for what total forgiveness looks like and how to experience total forgiveness in order to live a totally free and anointed life. He states simply, "The ultimate proof of total forgiveness takes place when we sincerely petition the Father to let those who have hurt us off the hook—even if they have hurt not only us, but also those close to us."[1]

The poignant example provided by the Genesis story of Joseph's suffering, betrayal, imprisonment, and defamation demonstrates the godly strength and character that can be forged in a forgiving heart. Total forgiveness is a biblical principle. To be capable of it may at times seem impossible. Yet to forgive the assaults that we suffer at the hands of others is a necessity for our inner well-being. God admonishes us, "If you forgive men their trespasses, your heavenly Father will also forgive you. But if you do not forgive men their trespasses, neither will your Father forgive your trespasses" (Matt. 6:14–15).

To live in alignment with God, which brings inner peace, we must be willing to offer total forgiveness toward all those who have harmed or hurt us. Our communion with God will empower us to possess a disposition of joy that can see us through the most hurtful situation. His love will impart to us a spirit of reconciliation, which is full of mercy toward others, just as God is merciful toward us.

Forgiveness is the only path to inner healing when we have been wronged; otherwise resentment and bitterness will corrupt our heart and refuse to allow us the peace of a forgiving heart. Outstanding grudges and grievances can only cause or facilitate anger, illness, and despondency. Depression and a festering vengefulness will drag us into darkest despair. A human spirit bound in such a manner does not allow the Father to teach or the Holy Spirit to anoint. There is no healing, then, in a heart filled with the malice and ill will that arise out of unforgiveness.

There is, of course, an additional dimension to forgiveness that affects our inner healing. That is the need to receive forgiveness for our own mistakes, for the wrongs we have committed before God's eyes. Accepting God's forgiveness for wrongs we have done to others and asking their forgiveness is as vital to our spiritual healing as our being able to forgive.

Dr. James Avery, a hospice physician, makes the observation that those who are dying often have huge regrets in their life revolving around a lack of receiving or giving forgiveness. Unforgiveness is an immense spiritual weight, and there can be no healing until that weight is laid aside. Dr. Avery has a prescription for people who are struggling with unforgiveness during the process of dying, which he borrowed from another hospice physician, Ira Byock. The prescription is based on the biblical principle for forgiveness; it is simply a list of five things to say to loved ones:

- Please forgive me.
- I forgive you.
- Thank you.
- I love you.
- Good-bye.[2]

Human nature is sinful. We must actively seek forgiveness from those we have hurt and, more, from God for hurting others whom He loves. Forgiveness is a necessary precondition to inner healing. The intellectual aspects of sin—which involve the mental (and perhaps physical) manifestations of sin—lead to depression and illness. These shadows not only prevent a process of healing, they are the antithesis—the opposite—of any healing. The intellectual aspects of sin and their inner illnesses can only be eliminated by an appeal to God's grace, which He is very willing to give, for strength to forgive.

The importance of being able to forgive and of being forgiven—by God and other people—cannot be underestimated in the process of our inner healing. Living in the state of a lack of forgiveness of others is a great obstacle that makes healing impossible, as I mentioned. It is pride, again, that does not allow us to ask for or offer forgiveness, receive our healing, and assist in the healing of others. God will give us grace to humble ourselves to the posture of forgiveness and to be set free from the bondage unforgiveness brings to our entire being.

DON'T LOSE YOUR ANOINTING

It is rare to meet an individual who has not been hurt by another human being through betrayal, abuse, or some form of injustice. From childhood, we sense the unfairness of treatment we receive from others, whether family, teachers, friends, employers, or a significant other. When we suffer injustice, we can submit our pain to God, and in that place of communion with Him we can receive His rest and the peace of His redemption, trusting in His promises as the psalmist did.

> I will wait for You, O You his Strength; for God is my
> defense....I will sing of Your power; yes, I will sing
> aloud of Your mercy in the morning; for You have
> been my defense and refuge in the day of my trouble.
> —PSALM 59:9, 16

Mean-spirited retaliation is not an option when we suffer an injustice done to us. Rather, we need to focus our minds on God and ask for the grace to love our enemies, as His Word commands us to do. (See Matthew 5:43–45.) When we call on the Lord and thank Him daily for helping us to live free from the sins of bitterness, anger, wrath, and revenge, He will give us grace to forgive our enemies.

When we are wounded and perplexed by injustice, especially those wounds inflicted by friends and family, it is imperative that we maintain our inner focus on our love relationship with our Lord. If we have learned that the priority of life as God intended it is to live in the mystery of divine romance with Him, nothing must be allowed to separate us from our Beloved.

When my friend R. T. Kendall leaves my home at the end of a visit, he always says to me, "Don't lose your anointing." I am grateful for the reminder. The anointing, that tangible presence of the glory of Christ in me, must be treasured and guarded continually. I must not allow anger, resentment, unforgiveness, or any other sin to quench the sweet anointing of the Holy Spirit. It is imperative that I determine to forgive others so I don't grieve the Holy Spirit (Eph. 4:30). When I suffer injustice at the hands of another person, I need to pray for a conciliatory attitude; in that prayer I know I will receive grace to bless my offender.

One practical consideration for blatant disregard for your well-being: Regardless of your station in life you should expect people to treat you justly. If they do not, you may confront them kindly and attempt to bring peace to the situation. If they are not willing to resolve the situation and there is just cause, you may need to allow the legal system to intervene. For example, situations of child abuse or spousal abuse often need professional intervention for reasons of safety. Yet even in such challenging times it is imperative that you pray for your enemies and receive grace from God to love them. That is the secret to inner healing and health, to really being at peace in the most challenging situations where people try to take advantage of you or those you love.

FORGIVENESS IS A NEW TESTAMENT MANDATE

Christ's atonement is not only the remedy for our personal sin but also the remedy for our inability to forgive those who sin against us. His supernatural grace empowers us to forgive the ones who hurt us most deeply. As we commune with Him, we are filled with His grace. Then we are able to choose to forgive those who have sinned against us. He empowers us to become an intercessor for the offending party, not an accuser, as we discussed earlier. (See chapter 3.) It is important to know the Scriptures say that where Christ is, seated at the right hand of the Father, He ever lives to make intercession for us (Heb. 7:25). One of the most Christlike qualities we can demonstrate is to pray for those who treat us unjustly.

Do you remember what Christ spoke from the cross? He cried out, "Father, forgive them, for they do not know what they do" (Luke 23:34). It is humanly impossible to understand the great love Jesus expressed toward His murderers in that prayer. Yet when Christ truly dwells within you, you can

expect His love in your heart to respond to your worst enemies in that same way.

We discussed the power of unforgiveness to cause unhealth
earlier. It is imperative that you understand that unforgiveness works more destruction in your own soul than it does
harm to your enemy. That is because unforgiveness breaks
your fellowship with the Lord and prevents your receiving all
the forgiveness you need for peace with God. R. T. Kendall
explains that when you choose to release your enemies from
your unforgiveness, you are the one who will be set free.

> When everything in you wants to hold a grudge,
> point a finger, and remember the pain, God wants
> you to lay it all aside. You can avoid spiritual quick-
> sand and experience the incredible freedom found in
> total forgiveness.[3]

Jesus asked the searching question, "For if ye love them
which love you, what thank have ye? for sinners also love
those that love them" (Luke 6:32, KJV). Jesus gave this mandate filled with promise: "But love ye your enemies, and do
good, and lend, hoping for nothing again; and your reward
shall be great, and ye shall be the children of the Highest: for
he is kind unto the unthankful and to the evil. Be ye therefore
merciful, as your Father also is merciful" (vv. 35–36, KJV).

In *Pilgrim's Progress*, John Bunyan's classic allegory of the
Christian life, Christian (the pilgrim) experienced release from
a heavy load when he came up on the cross on his journey
to the Celestial City.[4] He was released from the burden of the
world around him. Forgiveness of others brings a freedom very
much like the lifting of a heavy load off our back. In forgiving
our enemies, we are freed from carrying the harmful emotional load of retaliation, bitterness, and anger that threatens
to destroy our souls.

FORGIVING THE WORST

Chuck Colson, author of *How Now Shall We Live?*, discusses alternative options we have when we need to forgive another person.[5] He asks the reader to consider how he or she would respond to a person who committed a heinous crime, such as molesting and killing their child. He suggests three possible reactions:

1. Seek revenge and kill the perpetrator.

2. Seek justice through the judicial system.

3. Seek out the person, invite him into their home, forgive him, and offer him an inheritance in their estate.

What caring human being could *naturally* offer forgiveness to a criminal who killed his or her child? The natural reaction would be to kill the criminal in revenge. A restrained response would be to seek legal justice for the crime committed. While that may be required by the legal system, your personal response will necessarily be to seek the infinite grace of God to forgive this enemy who has inflicted such loss on your family. God will be faithful to give you His supernatural empowerment to become an intercessor for this sinner, who desperately needs to know the love of God.

Colson cites this horrendous example of tragic injustice to show the magnitude of what Christ did for every sinner when He died on Calvary for our sin. He came to the earth to seek and to save men and women who sinned against God and against their neighbors. Set in this tragic human scenario, we can recognize how impossible our task is to forgive our enemies as God forgave us. We understand that forgiveness is truly a divine grace that can only be experienced in that place of communion with our Lord, where He can minister healing to your broken heart.

God's great, loving heart forgave every heinous act committed by mankind against Him. He offers to give sinners who repent an inheritance in His kingdom of love. Such grace is unfathomable, divine, and entirely supernatural. As the Scriptures declare, "Ye know the grace of our Lord Jesus Christ, that, though he was rich, yet for your sakes he became poor, that ye through his poverty might be rich" (2 Cor. 8:9, KJV).

One of the greatest reasons we must determine to press into the rest of God (Heb. 4) is that we do not have the power in ourselves to forgive our enemies. While there is nothing in human nature that can conquer bitterness, resentment, or the desire for revenge, Jesus' command to love our enemies remains. (See Luke 6:27–28, 35.) And He does not give us a command that He will not give us His grace to fulfill as we surrender to His love.

WHAT FORGIVENESS IS NOT

In order to be able to forgive effectively, it is important to understand what forgiveness is *not*. R. T. Kendall explains that forgiveness is not a *feeling*; it is a *choice* you make.[6] In humble dependence on the supernatural grace of God you choose to allow His divine love to flow through you toward your enemy. Having said that, to remove confusion that hinders us from forgiving, we also need to know what forgiveness is *not*. It is not:

- approving what they did

- excusing what they did

- justifying what they did

- pardoning what they did—for example, a criminal must pay his debt to society

- reconciliation—this requires the participation of two people
- denying what they did
- blindness to what happened
- forgetting what they did
- refusing to take the wrong seriously
- pretending we are not hurt[7]

God never approves, excuses, or justifies sin; He recognizes it for what it is and then chooses to forgive based on His infinite divine love through the atonement of Christ. True forgiveness means being aware of the wrong and yet choosing to keep no record of it, refusing to punish, and relinquishing all bitterness and resentment toward your enemy—by the grace of God. When you make that choice, the Holy Spirit empowers you to truly forgive, and then He floods your soul with His peace and joy.

Forgiveness is a divine inner heart condition that responds to your enemy in mercy and gentleness through the grace of God. When it seems impossible to your human mind that you would be able to forgive a deep hurt inflicted on you by another, let your faith in God's love help you appropriate the wonderful promise of God's grace as found in 2 Corinthians 12:9–10.

We can have the supernatural power of God's grace for every kind of difficulty and distress. In your weakness, when you are tempted to harbor unforgiveness, His divine strength will help you to forgive. Receiving God's grace to forgive brings your soul into the supernatural rest of His love. In that place, the love of God will begin to supernaturally change your negative feelings toward those who have wronged you.

HOW TO KNOW WHEN YOU HAVE TOTALLY FORGIVEN

You may wonder how to know if you have totally forgiven those who betrayed you and altered your entire life through their unloving actions or words. R. T. Kendall writes that we will know when we have totally forgiven our enemies when we:

- don't tell others what they did to us
- don't let them fear us
- don't try to make them feel guilty
- let them save face
- protect them from their greatest fear (their sin being discovered)
- make forgiveness a lifelong commitment
- pray for them to be blessed[8]

Each of these propositions is important to understand and practice. For example, it is not possible to assume we have totally forgiven just because we did it one time. According to Kendall, we must make forgiving others a "life sentence."[9] We need to continually guard our hearts against the devil, who will look for ways to stir bitterness and resentment in our souls against others.

DISCUSSION 🌿 QUESTIONS

Do we have the power to forgive others who have wronged us? Can we forgive without receiving God's grace? Explain.

....

....

....

....

Does the Christian life need a continual source of anointing? Do we need to continually say to one another, "Don't lose your anointing"? Why or why not?

....

....

....

....

Which is more valid for a true Christian: becoming an intercessor or an accuser? Explain.

....

....

....

....

CHAPTER 7

FINDING
YOUR REST

T
O FULLY EXPERIENCE God's prescription for your inner healing, you need to have the touch of each person of the Trinity upon your soul. One of the characteristics of the triune God—the Father, Son, and Holy Spirit—is to be our Jehovah Rapha, the Lord our Healer. We must learn to rest in the healing bosom of the Trinity, where we find the essence of our spiritual healing.

We often begin our relationship with the great physician by coming to the Son of God as the only One who can forgive us. We realize that only His death on the cross can remove the penalty of our sins and grace us with the righteousness of God. To know this forgiveness is to extinguish the guilt that plagues us as well as to remove shame and a sense of rejection. We know that by being forgiven, we are cleansed and welcomed at the throne of God.

However, many people arrive at an understanding of the love of God as *Father* only after finding forgiveness through Christ. There may be things about your earthly parental upbringing that still cause you pain or skepticism. But God's Word has made it very clear that each one of us still needs parenting from the hand of God throughout our lives. You were created to have an inner longing for God the Father's acceptance and outpoured love. Even in the midst of illness and suffering, when you sense your limitations and disabilities, you can rejoice that the Father heart of God has purposed the trial you need in order to grow. He has promised to work everything for good (Rom. 8:28). He is God the Father Almighty, and His sovereignty teaches you to trust Him and to fear not. You can cast all your cares on Him because you know that He cares for you (1 Pet. 5:7). No beloved child will feel more secure or encouraged than the believing, forgiven child of God who knows how to rest in the Father heart of God.

The longer you live the Christian life in this world as it is, the more you will learn how much you need the Holy Spirit and how much your inner rest and health depend upon Him. Every Christian is called to serve others. The Lord Jesus declared that He "did not come to be served, but to serve" (Matt. 20:28). As disciples of Christ, that is to be our posture with our fellow man as well. It is laid out so plainly for us in Galatians 6:2: "Bear one another's burdens, and so fulfill the law of Christ." The same is found in Galatians 5:13: "Through love serve one another."

As you serve others, sometimes you will find that they do not always appreciate your efforts. There will be times you need healing for the wounds that result from lack of appreciation for your efforts so that you do not become weary in well doing (Gal. 6:9). As you offer up your service to God first of all as a sacrifice to please Him, you will be consoled by the Holy Spirit. He will restore you to a place of rest and peace as you focus on living your life to please God. He is your audience of one for all you do. By living your life to please Him, you will often subsequently be pleasing His people also.

In your service to others there will also be times when you feel the pain of watching others persist in self-destructive behaviors that destroy themselves or their families. You cannot change another person's heart if that person does not desire to change. The Holy Spirit is the power of God, who in answer to prayer can change the heart of stone into a heart of flesh. He can bring reconciliation when all your efforts have failed. As you learn to rest in dependence upon the Holy Spirit's intervention, you will be able to persevere despite any discouragement you may feel. The Holy Spirit brings healing to the dejected servant of God who feels as if he has expended himself in vain.

The Spirit also restores His rest to your soul when you fall into spiritual decline—when the Scriptures do not speak to you as they did and your prayers lack a sense of His presence. At times you may fear you have left your first love when you cannot seem to revive the freshness of your "springtime" communion with the Savior.

The prophet Isaiah said that when the Spirit is poured out from on high, He turns the wilderness into a fruitful field (Isa. 32:15). He pours out upon the dry ground of the thirsty (Isa. 44:3). He revives us again so that we may rejoice in Him (Ps. 85:6). This spiritual healing is available to every true child of God who is grieved by his or her own backsliding heart and who is unsatisfied with lack of communion with Him.

This healing work of the Holy Spirit in your inner man is a wonderful part of the experiential side of salvation. He becomes in you "a fountain of water springing up into everlasting life" (John 4:14). He becomes a river of water flowing through your innermost being (John 7:37–39). The Spirit of God fills you, revives you, and renews you. He anoints you with His own gracious presence to give you a lively faith that sees this life in light of eternity. You will learn to live a life marked for eternity in the present moment.

Your spiritual healing is also dependent upon your finding your anointed purpose in a God-centered and others-centered lifestyle. All human nature tends to be plagued with feelings of insignificance and uselessness. The antidote to these feelings is an awareness of God's anointed purpose for your life, which is conveyed to you by the blessed Spirit of God. To have an anointed purpose for life is one of the greatest rewards of life with God in the here and now.

Through your nature—the design of your heart, mind, and inner longing for communion with your Creator—you seek and are capable of receiving His divine rest for your soul, which is the essence of inner healing. God's twofold aspect of spiritual healing—forgiveness and a new life—are found in union with Christ through the cross. Through salvation He gives you a new heart, an anointed purpose, wholeness, and an eternal life of bliss in His presence—forever.

DISCUSSION ❧ QUESTIONS

List any obstacles in your life that have prevented you from aligning with God's prescription for inner healing.

....

....

....

....

Pray a prayer of repentance right now and ask God to help you remove those obstacles. Write anything you feel God is saying to you as you talk to Him in prayer.

....

....

....

....

Write a scripture that applies to your situation.

....

....

....

....

FOCUSING
ON ETERNITY

ALVATION THROUGH CHRIST gives our lives an entirely different focus, as we have discussed. When we are born again, receiving Christ's forgiveness for our sins, eternity lives in our hearts. And when you receive the blessing of eternity into your life, you begin to live with the same divinely ordained purpose for your life you will have for all eternity. Except for bringing souls to Christ, which is every Christian's mandate on earth, your God-given purpose to know God, glorify Him, and enjoy Him forever will characterize your life throughout eternity.

Within that eternal mandate, God gives us a special gifting and anointing to serve Him in practical ways as part of the body of Christ in the earth. You need to seek God to anoint you and equip you to live out the purpose for which He created you, with your eyes on Him. And you need to live continually in communion with Him for Him to show you how to fulfill that purpose.

For example, some are called by God to serve the church in leadership capacities, such as pastors or teachers. Others are commissioned to go to the nations as missionaries to bring the good news of Christ's salvation to those who have not heard. Many are called to be mothers and fathers who rear godly children and give to others in meaningful ways as God directs. Whether you sense a calling to a specific vocation or to simply living a godly life that will reflect the love of Christ in the earth, it is important that your focus is on eternal values.

For example, Christian physicians are able to render a service to people to promote healing for their bodies as well as love them in ways that will minister to their souls. Some patients, for example, go to doctors whom they know will spend time talking to them just because they need that sense of companionship and caring. That is a wonderful, beautiful characteristic of a person, no matter their vocation. Other patients simply want to receive the medical service you offer and then be on their way. Catering to both types of patients, doctors who are focused on eternity are living out the anointed purpose of their lives.

FACING THE TEMPORAL WITH THE PERSPECTIVE OF THE ETERNAL

Are you living your life preoccupied solely with the temporal, or are you focused on the eternal purpose for your life? Paul shows us his perspective of the hardships of this temporal life in light of his eternal focus.

> Therefore we do not lose heart. Even though our outward man is perishing, yet the inward man is being renewed day by day. For our light affliction, which is but for a moment, is working for us a far more exceeding and eternal weight of glory, while we do not look at the things which are seen, but at the things which are not seen. For the things which are seen are temporary, but the things which are not seen are eternal.
>
> —2 CORINTHIANS 4:16–18

Paul realized the temporal sorrows, trials, and afflictions that affected his outward man, which would one day perish, were working for his eternal good, actually preparing him for his eternal life that was to come. He is saying that these day-to-day afflictions are helpful to us if we continue to be focused on our eternal purpose. They make us humbler and bring us to renewed submission to God's will.

Through them we learn to say again and again, "Nevertheless not my will, but thine, be done" (Luke 22:42, KJV). These temporal trials compel us to seek God as our eternal comfort and portion in this life. Thus we are living more and more from the standpoint of eternity. Ask yourself, "How will this trial help me to live for eternity?" God sees and delights to reward the faithfulness of His children during their trials. This will make heaven more glorious.

Paul learned to live with a distinct spiritual gaze and focus apart from the trials he faced in this life. He aligned his soul in the direction of eternity. He admonishes us not to focus on the things seen but to give our positive consideration to the things that are unseen. Keep looking at the unseen, or you will become discouraged. Don't be easily distracted and thereby lose focus on your intimate relationship with God, the source of your rest and inner health.

When you worry, covet, or fear, you are fixated on the earthly side of things and will lose sight of God's eternal purposes for your life. Lose your focus, and you will lose sight of God's goodness and intervening power. Doing so will take you away from serving Him in joy and worshipping Him alone. When you look on the eternal things, you will keep focused on God and His rule over all. Keep your eyes on Jesus, and fellowship with Him in the midst of your disappointments and sorrows. A focus like this will strengthen you and enable you to go forward with God.

To keep from being easily distracted, you must remember as Paul did that what you see is temporal; what you don't see is eternal. It requires faith to contemplate eternity. Our future with God is forever. Ask yourself, "Which is most important for me to focus on, the cares of this life or the glory of God as His servant and worshipper and friend?" The Scriptures teach us to cast our cares on Him and to rejoice always; that is an eternal perspective of temporal life.

MOTIVATED BY HOPE OR DESPAIR?

When Paul says that we do not lose heart, he shows that the believer's motivation is filled with hope because our focus is different from those who seek after only what is seen—the temporal. Paul references two different motivations for facing life. First, he acknowledges the despair of our outward man, our body, which is perishing (2 Cor. 4:16). If we adopt that perspective, we will focus entirely on what we see with our eyes and experience in our natural man (v. 18).

However, there is a second motivation for facing life that fills our hearts with hope—it is our focus on pleasing God, and that will be rewarded in eternity. The reward we receive when we maintain this eternal focus is one of the weightiest rewards in glory (v. 17). With this eternal focus we will not lose heart in our temporal trials. Instead we are filled with hope, considering the eternal reality of the invisible, the hidden springs of God's Spirit, which are already present and working in our lives. We look to the Savior, who is interceding for us at the right hand of God, and we walk in the peace and rest He came to give us. In the final analysis one who pursues eternal realities receives more in this life as well as in eternity than those who forfeit their eternal blessing by choosing to focus on the temporal life.

In summary, the promise of living eternally in heaven with our Lord is a reward of ultimate healing for all of our illnesses, both physical and spiritual. Therefore, it is a message of hope. Hope looks forward with expectation to the good that God has promised us—eternally. Hope is joined to joy in Scripture (e.g., "rejoicing in hope" in Romans 12:12). Hope possesses in advance that which is yet to come. Our hearts can sing when they are full of hope, even in the face of painful situations.

The patient with this eternal hope has the foundational disposition for the healing of his inner man and is predisposed to activate all of the body's natural resources that enhance healing. Paul describes this hope as an active grace spurring him more and more toward an eternal perspective for all of life. We can follow his example and allow the Holy Spirit to fill our hearts with this hope as we embrace an eternal perspective of life.

In a very practical way Paul was saying this: it is natural to look at pain, rejection, discouragement, and setbacks. But in the face of those temporal things that are seen, Paul said he focused on eternal things: God's hand at work; God's promised goodness in His Word; the work of the Spirit within us to sanctify us by our trials; and the goodness of God to give us the privilege to serve Him and be His ambassadors.

He also kept in mind that every ounce of spiritual strength he received was obtained for him by the Savior's work on the cross. It was sent down from heaven as the fruit of the Savior's intercession in heaven on our behalf. He saw himself enveloped by the constant activity of the triune God for him, in him, and on his behalf. His benediction for each day of his life was this: "The grace of the Lord Jesus Christ, and the love of God, and the communion of the Holy Spirit be with you all. Amen" (2 Cor. 13:14).

If you live by the principles given to you in Paul's exhortation that we discussed, the following powerful truths will be written on your heart:

- Your life is one of hope; you do not lose heart.
  Your life is marked by what is strengthened,
  glorious (you are working at something that
  will be glorious), and forever.

- Your life is one of mystery in that your help
  is invisible, unseen, and nourished by hidden

springs in the soul. Therein lie your strength and confidence.

- Your life is one of contradiction and paradox. The paradox is that the greatest part of your life is the unseen part of life. A progressive strengthening and aim for glory are going on in the midst of your life on earth, which seems full of contradictions and trials because your outward man is perishing.

- Your life as a believer is one that is eternal. It will not end. Your trials will be long forgotten one day. As John Wesley reminds us, "The things that are seen [are] men, money, things of earth. The things that are not seen [are] God, grace, heaven."[1] Where is your focus? Where is the alignment of your heart?

God's eternal purpose for the redemption of your soul includes the healing of your body as well as your mind and spirit. He wants you to experience His love in such a way that you enjoy inner healing and health during your journey through life in His redemption. In these pages I have tried to encourage you to recognize the obstacles that will hinder that perfect rest and wholeness God has provided for you to enjoy in your intimate relationship with Him. The remedies for those obstacles have proven to bring healing to those who put their faith in Christ and the work of the Holy Spirit in their lives, and the grace of God provides you with power to effect those remedies. God teaches you through His Word and in your worshipful communion with Him to alter your focus from your temporal concerns to an eternal perspective filled with God's promises and purposes for your life.

My prayer for you, dear reader, will continually be that of Paul, which is for all believers.

I bow my knees to the Father of our Lord Jesus Christ...that He would grant you, according to the riches of His glory, to be strengthened with might through His Spirit in the *inner man*, that Christ may dwell in your hearts through faith; that you, being rooted and grounded in love, may be able to comprehend with all the saints what is the width and length and depth and height—to know the love of Christ which passes knowledge; that you may be filled with all the fullness of God.

—EPHESIANS 3:14, 16–19, EMPHASIS ADDED

DISCUSSION ⚘ QUESTIONS

As you focus on your eternal consummation with God, are you able to rest more in His redemption? Explain.

....

....

....

....

Why is it important that our relationship with Christ be the source of great joy?

....

....

....

....

Is our eternal friendship with the Creator the greatest relationship available to us? Can we achieve this eternal friendship without the mystery and romance of abandoning ourselves to His grace, His love, and His redemption? Explain.

....

....

....

CHAPTER 9

UNVEILING YOUR
NEW HEART

A S THIS BOOK comes to a close, may all who read it embrace the message and want to pursue the application of it to your life and thinking and practice. Some of you may want to read it one more time just to let it sink in, just to pray as you read and say, "Blessed Savior, work this in me more and more."

So in one sense we have finished presenting this message of inner healing through relationship with God in the previous chapters. But in another sense you may be one who wants to linger longer at the mercy seat of God's presence and have a new day's mercies poured out in your heart. For that reader we say again, there is nothing as powerful for your inner healing and health as living in communion with the Father, Son, and Holy Spirit. The following application of the message of this book is meant to encourage you in your pursuit of that intimate communion with the Lord and to emphasize the priority it should have in your life.

When you have the life of God within you, which is achieved in union with the Son of God, you will be able to say, like Paul, "I live; yet not I, but Christ liveth in me" (Gal. 2:20, KJV). You become a partaker of the divine nature (2 Pet. 1:4). That is the life of God in the soul of man—in your soul!

It is called the seed of God within us (1 John 3:9). This principle of new life is permanent and stable; it does not waver or wither. It is wrought in you by the Holy Spirit at the new birth (John 3:3). The spiritual signs of the regenerate soul contrast markedly with a natural life principle that is probably more familiar to us.

SPIRITUAL VS. NATURAL

Natural life exists in the realm of the senses. The inclinations and tendencies that arise from the senses exist in a wide variety among humans. Some people may take interest in religious things as a result of their education or because they have fond memories of their upbringing. Others may be drawn to religion by curiosity or intellectual engagement. Some seek the approval and social commendation that may accompany a "religious" life. Others are motivated by respect for Christian character qualities such as virtue and moral justice. These natural tendencies are not bad in themselves; rather, they simply cannot be confused with a living relationship with God.

In comparison, the divine life within us consists in faith, which produces four branches: love for God, charity to men, purity, and humility. It is Christ who provides the pattern for this life of God in the soul of man. In Him we see all these qualities exemplified—expressed in their clearest, crystalline form.

The Lord Jesus demonstrates love to God in constant devotion, prayer, and communion with Him. The fire of delight was never extinguished in Jesus, and He remained diligent in doing His Father's will, even to death. Jesus shows us what true love for people is in His unbounded charity, patience with His enemies, and ultimate self-sacrifice. Christ remained pure, never falling out of alignment by seeking sinful pleasures. And the Son of God said to us, "Learn of me; for I am meek and lowly in heart" (Matt. 11:29, KJV). He demonstrated the reality of this attitude when He knelt to wash His disciples' feet after the last supper. (See John 13:3–5.)

When we discover the character of God, we discover that He is exactly who He claims to be. Our deep assurance of that is our faith, which gives rest to the soul, brings everything into alignment with Him, enabling the growth of the soul. This faith originates in looking at Jesus' death on the cross, His pardon for our sins, and His example.

The character of God will be seen in your life if you truly love God and express your love in prayer and worship. Adherence to His will follows as the true delight of your soul. Worship and service to God become delights to your new heart. Humbleness before God and others is expressed in the new, free-flowing, self-moving principle of life. Then love— love for God and love for one's fellow humans—is the summary and apex of your new life of resting in His redemption.

LOVE

There is an exchange of hearts in love. In that exchange you are refreshed and enlivened by the joy God possesses and the delight He shows in you. God's love to you far exceeds the love you can offer Him, yet even the tears of repentance and its sorrows have a sacred sweetness when you pour them out before the divine Beloved. Once your soul finds its satisfaction in God, then you can live from the strength of that felicity. You are renewed and healed.

Your love of others becomes an overflow of this love and delight in God. If you start at the wrong place and do not seek love and satisfaction in God first, you will experience perpetual frustration because no human being can bring this satisfaction. When God Himself is your first love and chief portion, then you have overflowing joy and love to channel to others, independently of their appreciation. This is the new life! This relationship with God is the fountain of refreshment for your spiritual life and the well from which you must draw your motives for living. When you know the nature and reality of your new life and how to nourish and revive it in love, you then will know how to perpetually find restoration and wholeness. This is the health of the soul!

The essence of being healed spiritually and living life anew is in a retreat from loving self toward loving God. Love is your delight in God Himself, beyond His gifts. Everyone desires forgiveness and an escape from hell to heaven, but heaven without Jesus is no salvation. Love is not a deed. Love is a reflex of the newly born heart responding to the beauty of God in Christ. A deed of love can be imitated, but a reflex of the heart cannot be. Love arises from the cell of the heart to the beauty of God in Christ. To truly love God, we must delight in a relationship with God that satisfies. Loving God is delighting in, cherishing, savoring, treasuring, revering, and admiring God beyond any gift—life and health notwithstanding. When we truly love God with all of our hearts, independently of our requests and expectations and above our own needs, then we will find satisfaction, meaning, and purpose.

Loving God is our state of awe, contentment, and tranquility in an existence next to Him. This is resting in the bosom of the Trinity. It is resting in His redemption. It is to have Him and not need anything else.

THE PURPOSE OF OUR LIVES AND ETERNITY

The inner healing found through the new life—the life of God in one's soul—is ultimately expressed in an anointed purpose. There is the deepest richness associated with an anointed purpose in your life because it has an impact now and for eternity.

The meaning of the anointed life can be seen in the life of King David in the Old Testament. David had a special anointing from God. He had made nearness to God his primary goal in life and consequently became the greatest king of Israel.

The anointed life means asking God to anoint everything you do rather than attempting to live by your own strength. This leads to an epiphany of your purpose. The anointed life is, in essence, being a real Christian rather than superficially practicing a religion. This added significance of life, meaning in life, and love in life is only found when you ask for the anointing and receive the anointing in Christ. Then life has real purpose.

The anointing of a purpose makes your life in the present more meaningful, more productive, and more passionate. You develop as a person and accomplish things to a far greater degree than would be possible from your own strength alone.

There is a beautiful eternal significance to this anointed purpose of life. This is the reward of a godly life. Scripture confirms it.

> But without faith it is impossible to please Him, for he who comes to God must believe that He is, and that He is a rewarder of those who diligently seek Him.
> —HEBREWS 11:6

> And behold, I am coming quickly, and My reward is with Me, to give to every one according to his work.
> —REVELATION 22:12

Your responsibility is huge: your mindset now will be your mindset in eternity. Where are you focused? Do you sense your life has a purpose? Is your life meaningful? Will it be? It all begins with Jesus' call to you in Matthew 11:28, "Come to Me, all you who labor and are heavy laden, and I will give you rest."

The anointed purpose of life in Christ gives meaning now and for eternity. Everything you do in life will be evaluated by the Lord when you stand before Him in glory. He not only enables you to live faithfully for Him here on earth, but He also will reward you in heaven for doing so. His Word clearly describes the path of life that brings blessing and reward: "You will show me the path of life; in Your presence is fullness of joy; at Your right hand are pleasures forevermore" (Ps. 16:11). Spiritual blindness keeps us from perceiving His best for us. The Holy Spirit is yours, and He reveals the seemingly hidden diamonds of truth if you prayerfully search the Scriptures for understanding. All the criteria for blessing and reward are present in God.

Those who reject the Lord in this life will be judged and receive eternal judgment according to that life here on earth. Those who have received Jesus as their Lord and Savior will also be judged for every thought, word, deed, and action done here on earth. In the New Testament, Paul understood this judgment and pleaded with the church to see life from an eternal perspective. The believers who had spiritual blind spots often missed Paul's challenge, as had the disciples when Jesus preached the Sermon on the Mount, recorded in Matthew.

Paul, well aware of God's grace, knew what it meant to be brought before a court of law and judged for one's actions. In the Greek city of Corinth his enemies dragged him into court for preaching the gospel. Scholars believe that a raised marble platform still visible today in the ruins of Corinth was the place where Paul's case was tried. The platform was referred to as the *bēma*, which is the Greek word for *judgment seat*. The *bēma* represented authority, justice, and reward. Later Paul sent a letter to the church in Corinth and spoke of another *bēma* in heaven (2 Cor. 5:10)—the judgment seat for Christians and the great white throne for nonbelievers.

You will be evaluated by how you behave during your time here on earth (your imaginations) and rewarded accordingly. Spiritual sight for the believer, your inner health, is achieved by an eternal desire to live today with eternity's values in view. And God's eternal reward system is extravagant!

Where you spend eternity is determined by belief: "Believe on the Lord Jesus Christ, and you will be saved" (Acts 16:31). How you spend eternity is determined by your faithfulness: "Well done, good and faithful servant! You have been faithful with a few things; I will put you in charge of many things. Come and share your master's happiness!" (Matt. 25:23, NIV).

To be anointed is to have meaning, direction, and purpose

that God appoints, prepares, superintends, and revives along the way. It is the interpenetration of God's Spirit and yours. You are thus equipped so that you are not left to yourself. You are infiltrated with the Most High, for whom nothing is impossible. Anointing is God saying, "I have chosen you, and I am going to be with you!" Our spiritual healing and physical health and wholeness derive from the harmony, joy, completeness, and anointed purpose in our alignment with God.

TWO PENETRATING INSIGHTS

The Savior has many penetrating insights into the real center of life that are recorded in the four Gospels. They refer to true satisfaction and the nature of the divine healing of which we all stand in need. Two of these insights provide a focus on inner healing for us here.

The first insight concerns what Jesus called the "one thing [that] is necessary"—namely to sit at His feet and to feed on His Word and His person. (See Luke 10:38–42, AMP.) While Martha bustled with the details of her hospitality for Jesus when He came to visit her home, her sister, Mary, sat at Jesus' feet and listened to His word.

"Martha was distracted with much serving, and she approached Him and said, 'Lord, do You not care that my sister has left me to serve alone? Therefore tell her to help me'" (v. 40). Jesus answered her with gentle admonishment, "Martha, Martha, you are worried and troubled about many things. But one thing is needed, and Mary has chosen that good part, which will not be taken away from her" (vv. 41–42).

For you to receive all the good that the great physician has in store for you, you must choose "that good part." You must sit at Jesus' feet daily and learn from Him the joy of His fellowship, the wisdom of His design for your life, and His anointed purpose for your life. What do you feed your soul— God's Word or your own worries? The Son of God speaks very personally to each of us: "It is written, 'Man shall not live by bread alone, but by every word that proceeds from the mouth of God'" (Matt. 4:4). The question you must ask yourself each day is this: Am I going to be a Mary today and sit at Jesus' feet, taking Him in, or am I going to be a distracted and burdened Martha instead?

Martha's actions in the account were founded on self-reliance and therefore were full of frustration. Mary's alternative of communion with her Lord and delighting in His presence represents a life full of satisfaction and contentment. In contrast to the busyness that Martha hoped would be generous to her guests, Mary's way generates a spirit permeated with the Lord, which provides us the best preparation for serving others.

The second insight derived from a crucial passage from the Gospels is found in Matthew in the parable of the treasure hidden in the field (Matt. 13:44). Jesus taught through the parable that the tendency to pursue one thing after the other—in a ceaseless search for the satisfaction of desire—inevitably ends in frustration and disappointment. In Jesus' allegory a certain man stumbled upon a treasure hidden in a field. Overcome with joy, he sold all that he possessed so he could buy the field. Jesus is the treasure hidden in the field—we must choose Him with passion as the only thing worth having. We will count it a joy to abandon all else as the source of our meaning when we find our all in all in Him. As long as we have Him, we will be rich and full and satisfied. This must be healing, or nothing is!

Jesus is the Shepherd who will guide you to green pastures and beside still waters. He is the King who by His power transforms your disappointments in life into something good (Rom. 8:28). He is the heavenly Bridegroom who fills you with the love of heaven. He is the Captain of your salvation who will lead you to be more than a conqueror. When He is yours, you can say, even in your weakest moments, that He is your strength. Jesus says to us, as He did to Paul: "My grace is sufficient for you, for My strength is made perfect in weakness" (2 Cor. 12:9). May you respond as the apostle did: "Therefore most gladly I will rather boast in my infirmities, that the power of Christ may rest upon me.... For when I am weak, then I am strong" (vv. 9–10). This is why Paul could say, "By the grace of God I am what I am, and His grace toward me was not in vain; but I labored more abundantly than they all, yet not I, but the grace of God which was with me" (1 Cor. 15:10).

The grace of God enables you to fulfill the anointed purpose for your life, through your experiences of illness and breakdown and into healing and health. Paul interpreted the disposition of spiritual vitality as "rejoice always, pray without ceasing, in everything give thanks" (1 Thess. 5:16–18). By such a life you may receive the grace of God daily, which empowers you to enjoy the restoration of your soul's health. Truly resting in His redemption brings you peace, and peace is "perfect well-being, all necessary good, all spiritual prosperity, and freedom from fears and agitating passions and moral conflicts" (2 Pet. 1:2, AMPC). Anyone that can claim that peace is healed.

DISCUSSION 🌿 QUESTIONS

What does purpose mean to you?

....

....

....

....

Do you feel you know what the purpose is for your life? Explain.

....

....

....

....

How does knowing God and His love change the purpose for your life and bring you to a new level of wholeness?

....

....

....

....

....

NOTES

CHAPTER 1

1. *Merriam-Webster*, s.v. "rest," accessed February 13, 2019, http://www.merriam-webster.com/dictionary/rest.
2. Augustine, *Confessions* 1.1, 1.5.
3. *Westminster Shorter Catechism* 1, http://www.westminsterconfession.org/confessional-standards/the-westminster-shorter-catechism.php.
4. Blue Letter Bible, s.v. "*shabbath*," accessed February 14, 2019, https://www.blueletterbible.org/lang/lexicon/lexicon.cfm?Strongs=H7676&t=KJV; Blue Letter Bible, s.v. "*shabath*," accessed February 14, 2019, https://www.blueletterbible.org/lang/lexicon/lexicon.cfm?Strongs=H7673.
5. WordNet, s.v. "redemption," accessed February 15, 2019, http://wordnetweb.princeton.edu/perl/webwn?s=redemption.

CHAPTER 2

1. See, for example, Alan Fogel, "Emotional and Physical Pain Activate Similar Brain Regions," *Psychology Today*, April 19, 2012, https://www.psychologytoday.com/us/blog/body-sense/201204/emotional-and-physical-pain-activate-similar-brain-regions.
2. See, for example, Chris Woolston, "Illness: The Mind-Body Connection," Lifestyle and Wellness, updated March 6, 2003, https://web.archive.org/web/20030802180339/http://blueprint.bluecrossmn.com/topic/depills; "Breast Cancer and Depression," Artemis—Feature Article, November 2000, www.hopkinsbreastcenter.org/artemis/200011/feature7.html; and Chris Woolston, "Depression and Heart Disease," Ills & Conditions, updated March 26, 2003, https://web.archive.org/web/20030415213655/http://blueprint.bluecrossmn.com/topic/depheart.

3. "Mental Health: A Report of the Surgeon General," US Public Health Service, 1999, chapter 1, https://web.archive.org/web/20000303220041/www.surgeongeneral.gov/Library/MentalHealth/chapter1/sec1.html#mind_body.

4. William Collinge, "Mind/Body Medicine: The Dance of Soma and Psyche," HealthWorld Online, accessed February 15, 2019, http://www.healthy.net/Health/Article/Mind_Body_Medicine/1949.

5. Andrew B. Newberg, Eugene G. D'Aquili, and Vince Rause, *Why God Won't Go Away: Brain Science and the Biology of Belief* (New York: Ballantine Books, 2002).

6. Dutch Sheets, *Tell Your Heart to Beat Again* (Ventura, CA: Gospel Light, 2002), 20.

CHAPTER 3

1. Jerry Bridges, *Respectable Sins: Confronting the Sins We Tolerate* (Colorado Springs, CO: NavPress, 2007).

CHAPTER 4

1. Joni Eareckson Tada, *When Is It Right to Die?* (Grand Rapids, MI: Zondervan Publishing, 1992), 177.

2. Randolph C. Byrd, "Positive Therapeutic Effects of Intercessory Prayer in a Coronary Care Unit Population," *Southern Medical Journal* 81 (1998): 826, http://www.godandscience.org/apologetics/smj.html. According to Google Scholar, this article has been cited 1,100 times as of February 22, 2019.

3. Byrd, "Positive Therapeutic Effects of Intercessory Prayer in a Coronary Care Unit Population," 829.

4. Byrd, "Positive Therapeutic Effects of Intercessory Prayer in a Coronary Care Unit Population," 829.

5. John Donne, *Devotions Upon Emergent Occasions,* "Meditation XVII," 1624, http://www.ccel.org/ccel/donne/devotions.iv.iii.xvii.i.html.

6. See for example Linda K. George, "The Health-Promoting Effects of Social Bonds," accessed February 15, 2019, https://web.archive.org/web/20060504205318/http://www.cossa.org/linda%20george.pdf; Sophia P. Glezos, "Social Relationships, Connectedness, and Health: The Bonds That Heal," Summary of a Presentation by Lisa F. Berkman,

Harvard School of Public Health, May 22, 1997, https://web. archive.org/web/20060502090712/http://obssr.od.nih.gov/ Publications/SOCIAL.HTM.

7. N. Frasure-Smith and R. H. Prince, "The Ischemic Heart Disease Life Stress Monitoring Program: 18-Month Mortality Results," *Canadian Journal of Public Health* 11, no. S1 (May–June 1986), S46–20, https://www.researchgate.net/ publication/19635319_The_Ischemic_Heart_Disease_Life_ Stress_Monitoring_Program_18-Month_mortality_results.

CHAPTER 5

1. Usha Lee McFarling, "Doctors Find Power of Faith Hard to Ignore," December 23, 1998, www.tennessean.com/health/ stories.98/trends1223.htm.

2. Studies include the following titles: "Religion and Blood Pressure," "Religious Attendance and Survival," and "Religion and Immune Function." See H. G. Koenig, et al., "The Relationship Between Religious Activities and Blood Pressure in Older Adults," International Journal of Psychiatry in Medicine 28 (1998): 189–213, https:// web.archive.org/web/20031018090803/http://www. dukespiritualityandhealth.org/pastreports.html.

3. Harold G. Koenig, "Religion, Spirituality, and Health: The Research and Clinical Implications," *ISRN Psychiatry* (2012): 278730, https://www.ncbi.nlm.nih.gov/pmc/articles/ PMC3671693/.

4. Blue Letter Bible, s.v. "*thalpō*," accessed February 18, 2019, https://www.blueletterbible.org/lang/lexicon/lexicon. cfm?strongs=G2282.

5. Mother Teresa, *The Joy in Loving: A Guide to Daily Living*, comp. Jaya Chaliha and Edward Le Joly (New York: Penguin Books, 1996), April 4, https://books.google.com/ books?id=l40HSskC0S0C&pg.

6. Mother Teresa, as quoted in Vincent Canby, "Screen: Documentary About Mother Teresa," *New York Times*, November 28, 1986, https://timesmachine.nytimes.com/ timesmachine/1986/11/28/174386.html?pageNumber=78.

7. "Prayer and Intercession Quotes (1)," Tentmaker, accessed February 19, 2019, http://www.tentmaker.org/Quotes/prayerquotes.htm.

CHAPTER 6

1. R. T. Kendall, *Total Forgiveness* (Lake Mary, FL: Charisma House, 2002), 4.
2. Mary Faulds, "Life for the Dying," *AFA Journal* (November–December 2009), https://afajournal.org/past-issues/2009/november-december/life-for-the-dying/.
3. Kendall, *Total Forgiveness*, back cover.
4. John Bunyan, *Pilgrim's Progress* (Grand Rapids, MI: Christian Classics Ethereal Library, n.d.), 33, https://www.ccel.org/ccel/bunyan/pilgrim.pdf.
5. Charles W. Colson and Nancy Pearcey, *How Now Shall We Live?* (Wheaton, IL: Tyndale, 1999).
6. Kendall, *Total Forgiveness*, 21.
7. Kendall, *Total Forgiveness*, 11–19.
8. R. T. Kendall, *How to Forgive Ourselves Totally* (Lake Mary, FL: Charisma House, 2007), 175–176.
9. Kendall, *How to Forgive Ourselves Totally*, 175.

CHAPTER 8

1. John Wesley, "Commentary on 2 Corinthians 4:18," *John Wesley's Explanatory Notes on the Whole Bible*, accessed February 19, 2019, https://www.studylight.org/commentary/2-corinthians/4-18.html.

ABOUT THE
AUTHOR

J AMES P. GILLS, MD, received his medical degree from Duke University Medical Center in 1959. He served his ophthalmology residency at Wilmer Ophthalmological Institute of Johns Hopkins University from 1962 to 1965. Dr. Gills founded the St. Luke's Cataract and Laser Institute in Tarpon Springs, Florida, and has performed more cataract and lens implant surgeries than any other eye surgeon in the world. Since establishing his Florida practice in 1968, he has been firmly committed to embracing new technology and perfecting the latest cataract surgery techniques. In 1974, he became the first eye surgeon in the United States to dedicate his practice to cataract treatment through the use of intraocular lenses. Dr. Gills has been recognized in Florida and throughout the world for his professional accomplishments and personal commitment to helping others. He has been recognized by the readers of Cataract & Refractive Surgery Today as one of the top fifty cataract and refractive opinion leaders.

As a world-renowned ophthalmologist, Dr. Gills has received innumerable medical and educational awards and has been listed in The Best Doctors in America. As a clinical professor of ophthalmology at the University of South Florida, he was named one of the best ophthalmologists in America in 1996 by ophthalmic academic leaders nationwide. He has served on the board of directors of the American College of Eye Surgeons, the board of visitors at Duke University Medical Center, and the advisory board of Wilmer Ophthalmological Institute at Johns Hopkins University.

While Dr. Gills has many accomplishments and varied interests, his primary focus is to restore physical vision to patients and to bring spiritual enlightenment through his life. Guided by his strong and enduring faith in Jesus Christ, he seeks to encourage and comfort the patients who come to St. Luke's and to share his faith whenever possible. It was through sharing his insights with patients that he initially began writing on Christian topics. An avid student of the Bible for many years, he has authored numerous books on Christian living, with over nine million copies in print. With the exception of the Bible, Dr. Gills' books are perhaps the most widely requested books in the US prison system. They have been supplied to over two thousand prisons and jails, including every death row facility in the nation. In addition, Dr. Gills has published more than 195 medical articles and has authored or coauthored ten medical reference textbooks. Six of those books were best sellers at the American Academy of Ophthalmology annual meetings.

Did You Enjoy This Book?
We at Love Press would be pleased to hear from you if
God's Rx for Inner Healing
has had an effect on your life or the lives of your loved ones.
Send your letters to:
Love Press
P.O. Box 1608
Tarpon Springs, FL 34688-1608